cancer

cancer

what they
don't
tell you
and what
you need
to know

Leigh Bernhardt

Published by Leigh Bernhardt

First published 2020

© 2020 Leigh Bernhardt

Disclaimer

The author does not profess to have any medical qualifications and has based the content of this book on his personal experience and general knowledge. Any advice contained herein is not to be substituted for medical or legal advice.

The author is not responsible for any actions taken by any persons taken after reading this book and advises that in all cases medical advice be sought as required in relation to any illness, medical conditions, prescription and/or over the counter medication and products, medicine or treatment readers may be experiencing or using. The information and advice is not provided to suit any specific circumstances and is general in nature only. The reader must use their own enquiries to determine the validity and appropriateness of any advice contained herein. Reliance on any of the advice or information contained herein is solely at the reader's own risk.

NATIONAL LIBRARY OF AUSTRALIA — A catalogue record for this book is available from the National Library of Australia

ISBN: 978 0 6488568 0 1 (pbk)
       978 0 6488568 1 8 (ebk)

Designed and typeset by Helen Christie, Blue Wren Books

"You are the best project that you will ever work on."

Contents

Introduction

My Backstory

In early 2008 at the age of 55, I was diagnosed with multiple myeloma. My diagnosis came over the telephone on a Friday afternoon from my GP, following some recent tests for a swollen knee after a running race.

I was a competent runner, triathlete and tennis player and kept myself in good physical condition. A non-smoker, I had also not consumed any alcohol for 17 years until after chemotherapy treatments. (I'll go into this later.)

The GP advised me of the seriousness of this condition and said he had scheduled an appointment for me with a haematologist on Monday morning.

The haematologist explained that the condition was not multiple myeloma, but stage 4 non-Hodgkin lymphoma. It was in some ways a relief, as this disease is generally more successfully treated than multiple myeloma, but it highlighted to me the potential for medical information to be incorrect and disturbing to the patient.

Following this diagnosis, I commenced a regime of chemotherapy treatments involving chemicals that I was told were essential to treat the disease but that had serious, and in some cases, permanent side effects.

The chemotherapy treatments continued for six months, followed by two years of maintenance infusions of a drug named MabThera, which helped stabilise the condition.

This drug sought out and identified the damaged white blood cells and destroyed them.

Each infusion at the time cost approximately $6,000, and I had about 10 infusions.

During the treatments, I suffered from the normal effects of chemotherapy such as hair loss, nausea, mouth ulcers, weight gain, swollen stomach, loss of taste and smell and peripheral neuropathy (loss of feeling in the extremities of the fingers and toes).

I also endured the side effects of the drugs used to combat the damage that chemotherapy can cause to other parts of the body during treatment, including steroids and pain medication.

Many of these side effects were not fully explained by the treating medical practitioners, who were focused principally on treating the disease, but their impact was profound at the time.

In 2011, I underwent a stem cell collection where I was given large doses of chemicals which destroyed my immune system so that new unaffected bone marrow and blood cells could be regenerated and harvested.

These stem cells were collected using an apheresis machine. Apheresis is a process where whole blood is removed from an individual and then separated into its components such as platelets and plasma, white and red blood cells.

It was a dramatic process and involved a great deal of discomfort, including sitting at the apheresis machine for up to five hours a day for a week in order to collect the required number of stem cells.

These stem cells remain frozen at my hospital in case I need them in the future for an autologous (self) transplant rather than having to rely on a donor.

The treatment was successful, and although the side effects of loss of taste and smell and the feeling in my extremities caused by the chemotherapy treatments remained, there was a period of approximately seven years of remission until 2018.

In 2017, after years of complaining of indigestion to my doctor and being prescribed medication to treat the indigestion, I suffered a heart attack with a 99% blockage in my obtuse marginal artery.

It was later disclosed that because I was fit and relatively healthy, with normal blood pressure, my heart had worked around the blockage until it became too severe. No one thought that I had coronary heart disease, so my symptoms were treated as indigestion.

A stent was inserted into the affected artery. Apart from cholesterol-lowering medication, this issue now appears to be under control.

In 2018, I was diagnosed with cancer in both kidneys and underwent partial nephrectomies (partial removal of both kidneys) in separate surgeries six months apart.

During this process, the diversity of medical opinion between specialists was highlighted. One opinion was to remove at least one kidney, and possibly both, with dialysis as a real option. Another was to attempt to carry out partial removal of both kidneys using robotics and keyhole surgery.

The second option was chosen, and after two complex and difficult surgeries, I have returned to relatively good health with almost normal kidney function.

I also underwent two total hip replacements and hernia repair surgeries between 2011 and 2017.

I have written this book to help people who are facing cancer or other life-threatening conditions deal with the many and varied decisions they must take to achieve the best outcome possible under their circumstances.

The navigation of medical opinions, treatments, medication and recovery methods can be so varied that it takes time and significant effort to obtain the required information, consider all the options and contributing factors and make clear and decisive decisions which must be in your best interests.

Quite often, medical practitioners and nursing staff are focused on so many tasks that things that are important to you are often overlooked until they become apparent or critical.

During my numerous treatments and medical procedures, I discovered that in order to survive I needed to take control of my treatments and medication, manage any advice given to me and make decisions based on outcomes and practical applications, rather than rely on swimming with the tide and hoping things turned out for the best.

This on occasion meant that I delivered clear and precise instructions to medical practitioners and nursing staff with no room for equivocation or ambiguity.

Throughout this book I will provide examples of these occurrences, and I will also provide tips that in my view are helpful and may assist you in your journey.

I am not a doctor, nor do I profess to have any medical qualifications whatsoever. I am, however, alive after suffering through two serious bouts of stage 4 cancer, a heart attack and numerous surgeries.

Throughout these ordeals I have discovered that there are many ways to aid the treatment processes and to achieve better outcomes. Although much of this advice is out there in the system it does not always become available or known to the patient.

I have helped a number of friends and acquaintances with cancer and was able to provide useful and timely assistance during this stressful and anxious time of their lives. Their continued prompts to write about my experiences and the practical knowledge I have gained in order to help a wider audience instigated this book.

By reading this book, you have already achieved the main objective – staying alive.

We all will die of something sooner or later, so it is important to remember that cancer is a part of life for many people. The goal of staying alive and minimising collateral damage from medical interventions remains paramount.

With the often fantastic improvements in medicine continually being discovered and refined, survival rates, particularly for cancer, have risen dramatically. Recent statistics of worldwide survival rates demonstrate an increase from 50–67% (these are global figures averaged across all cancers, with some cancers having higher survival rates than others). The reasons for this increase in survivability of cancer-related illness is attributed in the main to the combination of early detection and improved treatment.

There is also significant evidence to support how a positive attitude, diet and exercise and tailored recovery strategies can dramatically improve outcomes related to these illnesses and associated treatments.

Throughout this book I constantly reinforce the advice that no matter how dire the diagnosis or the prognosis may be, a positive attitude tempered with a realistic assessment of the situation is essential to maximise the outcomes of the treatment, the management of your life in general and how you deal with future issues associated with your medical condition.

Chapter 1

The Diagnosis

It would be almost inhuman for a person to receive the diagnosis of a terminal or life-threatening illness without feeling apprehension, fear and uncertainty.

When this type of news is first delivered, the initial reaction is generally one of disbelief and anxiety.

Often the diagnosis is complex, and the treatment options and timeframes are outlined at this initial meeting.

Trying to concentrate on the discussion after the initial diagnosis is difficult, and it is easy to forget sections of the discussion and sometimes crucial information.

Tip Number 1

If possible, take a family member or support person to the meeting. Ask the permission of the medical practitioner to record the meeting. This helps when relaying the information to family or friends and ensures you have all the information delivered at the time. It also allows time to consider the details and your options.

Depending upon the seriousness of the diagnosis, the medical practitioner may provide a timeframe or estimation of your life expectancy with or without treatments.

These timeframes are generally based on broad statistics and do not consider many of the circumstances of the individual such as general health, efficacy of medication and treatments, recovery strategies and attitude of the patient.

It may also be necessary to seek the opinion of a specialist/s or even a second or third opinion before surgery or treatment commences.

Decisions need to be made when you are as calm as possible and able to consider the implications of options such as radical surgery as opposed to chemical/radiation treatments. In some cases, the option may be to wait and see, with regular scans or tests scheduled to keep track of the illness or tumour/s with appropriate intervention when required.

It is not unusual for medical opinions to be different. Researching your diagnosis and treatment options is useful but using online opinions as anything more than background information can be dangerous.

Tip Number 2

Once you have the initial diagnosis, research as much information as you can on treatment options, medication and associated side effects specific to your condition. Compile questions for your next visit to your treating medical practitioner.

Advising family, friends and acquaintances is difficult but necessary so that they can provide moral and physical support during the treatment/s you may be facing.

Until all the information including timeframes, options, possible outcomes and upcoming appointments for things such as scans, x-rays, biopsies, MRIs and CAT scans are determined, information on your condition can be relayed in parts as they occur.

Misdiagnosis is not uncommon, and it may be best to make sure of your diagnosis after the appropriate tests have been carried out and a treatment plan devised before you start advising family and friends.

If the diagnosis is delivered by a specialist, return to

your GP and seek their opinion on other possible treatment options, or specialists who may be suitable to treat your issues.

Quite often there are conflicting views held by specialists and other medical practitioners on treatment options and considerations such as keyhole surgery, robotics and some chemotherapy treatments. This reinforces the advice to research your diagnosis and have as much information as possible before you commence your treatment.

A friend of mine who was relatively young (48 at the time of diagnosis) was diagnosed with terminal throat cancer.

He was super fit, and the diagnosis was catastrophic for him and his family, so when his options were explained, with the preferred treatment being the surgical removal of his entire lower jaw, tongue and voice-box, they were as devastated as anyone would be.

I met with him on numerous occasions where we discussed my passage through the treatment options I had been involved with and his options as well. Eventually, he decided to forgo the surgery and have what remained left of his time with the best possible quality of life.

He pursued holistic treatments and a strict dietary and supplements regime including maintaining his physical fitness and mental state.

The use of meditation, yoga and other relaxation practices

kept him centred and focused on achieving all he could with his remaining time.

After approximately 12 months, he returned to the cancer specialist who had initially advised the radical surgery, and when he saw the state of his patient he commented that he was pleased that he had refused the surgery as his quality of life and life expectancy would have been far less than the outcome before him now.

My friend lived for approximately another year before succumbing to the disease, but he squeezed every drop of living out of his circumstances. Apart from a large growth on his throat he appeared normal, and was able to surf, run, eat and live just like anybody else.

This is just one example of the need to carefully consider your options and treatments so that all outcomes and consequences are on the table and the short- and long-term outcomes considered together.

Research and knowledge are important for you to understand the advice on your condition from the medical specialists providing your treatment and care, and to convey this information to family and carers.

Quite often, cancer sufferers become very knowledgeable about their condition by researching information and other cases related to their medical condition.

Cancer patients conducting research are focused on a very narrow field of medicine specific to their individual circumstances. They are therefore able to provide constructive contemporary details to their treating medical practitioners about medication and advancements in treatments which may be beneficial.

It is an often-forgotten fact that many doctors and nurses have never taken some of the drugs they prescribe, or experienced the after-effects of chemotherapy or surgery. Their knowledge is based on their training, advice and literature.

Only people who have taken chemotherapy drugs can really tell you how it makes them feel, and what side effects they suffered.

From my discussions with patients undergoing chemotherapy, although there are commonly known clinical outcomes, each person's reaction to drugs and the side effects they experience are acutely affected by issues such as the nature and stage of the cancer, age, health, fitness, mental attitude, treatment conditions and other contributing factors.

Seeking out someone who has undergone a similar treatment to what is proposed for you may assist with some of the problems you are about to face and provide some non-clinical but practical advice.

This includes the treatment and medicine available, possible treatment options and side effects.

Being able to discuss these matters with your treating

team allows discussion on the merits and downsides of some treatments and helps all parties understand your particular requirements.

Tip Number 3

Compile a file, including a notebook, to keep all your medical information in one place (one or more files) for easy access and reference. Download and record information to your PC for backup and place all electronic communications related to your medical issues in one place on your PC and on a backup hard drive if possible.

There is often a tendency to rush into commencing medication and/or treatments, especially when the diagnosis is dire.

Obviously, everybody's circumstances are different and everybody handles their emotions in different ways. However, because of the severity of the decisions to be made relating to your treatment and available options, if possible, take some time to discuss your views and concerns with family and friends, or go back to your local GP and cover off any uncertainties you may have.

It is vital that you have confidence in the treating surgeon/specialist/s conducting your treatment. If this confidence does not exist, then seek a referral to one or more other specialists until you are satisfied with the diagnosis and the treatment options.

Some indicators that may require you to consider such actions are where your treating specialist disregards your questions/concerns and does not consider your particular circumstances or requirements relative to your condition and treatment.

Statements such as 'we need to remove that growth as soon as possible' or 'we need to commence chemotherapy or radiation treatment immediately' should be met with enquiries such as:

- How will the surgery be performed and what other less invasive or dramatic options are available?
- What type of drugs are involved in the chemotherapy regime recommended, and what supplementary drugs are associated with this treatment and what are their side effects?
- Is my diagnosis confirmed based on the results of the tests performed to date or are there more exploratory or diagnostic options available before we commence treatment?
- What is the timeframe for commencement of my treatment including hospital stays and locations?
- What is the likely duration of my treatment?
- What is the estimated cost of the treatment and what

component of the treatment is claimable under either a government or private health fund (where applicable)?

- If I follow the treatment plan you have proposed, what is my prognosis after the treatment, whether successful or unsuccessful?
- What are my options and timeframes if, rather than proceeding immediately, I elect to adopt a wait and see option with regular scans and testing to monitor my condition?

Some of the things I was told were that some of the drugs I would be taking had significant adverse effects on my heart function and that a proportion of my heart muscle function might be irreparably damaged.

I was also informed that if I did not have the chemotherapy procedure, or I had it and it was not successful, I would probably not live for more than six months.

This is when the decisions become real and hard. As a strong, relatively fit athlete and part-time professional tennis coach, I was faced with a long period of sickness and possible loss of the ability to run, swim, play tennis and carry on life as before the diagnosis.

My ability to continue with my business as a human resources, industrial relations, mediation and commercial arbitration consultant and continue to earn an income would also be severely affected.

In the end, the decision for me was relatively simple: have the chemotherapy, understand the possible side effects and treat the whole process as a triathlon or race.

This meant undertaking a thought process that focused on:

- understanding the risks and the details of the event in order to successfully complete the event
- doing the required preparation and training
- having the best and most suitable equipment available
- having a good support team
- concentrating on my strengths and managing my weaknesses
- knowing that it would be tough, but being prepared for the ordeal
- giving up was not an option
- being around to run another race.

After the first round of chemotherapy drugs, I went to a cardiologist and had an exercise stress test on a treadmill and an echo cardiogram.

The results of those tests showed a 10–15% reduction in my heart function through damage to the heart muscle.

When I explained these results to the haematologist who was supervising my chemotherapy treatment, his answer was succinct and correct. "Don't go back to the heart specialist, because you need the chemotherapy and any damage caused by the chemotherapy is better than being dead."

I chose to continue with the chemotherapy infusions and associated medication.

They were sobering words and the cause of much distress at the time, however once I was in remission and back exercising regularly, I went back to the cardiologist for a repeat of the tests.

The results obtained two years after the first dose of chemotherapy was that my heart muscle had recovered to the extent that although some minor damage to the heart had occurred, in the words of the cardiologist there would be no discernible reduction in my ability to exercise, and I would be more likely to die from being hit by a bus than from heart failure.

These were ironic comments because at that stage there was no evidence of heart disease or cholesterol blockages, however I suffered a heart attack seven years later.

There is no doubt that my high level of fitness at the time and my history of athletic activity greatly improved my chances of survival and aided my recovery.

My history with diagnosis has been more luck than good management and once again my interventions and actions have definitively aided the process.

The non-Hodgkin lymphoma markers present in my blood tests for some time through increased eosinophils and anaemia were glossed over by my then GP as general inflammation. He apologised for not picking up on these symptoms once I was diagnosed by another GP.

The symptoms were only discovered when additional blood tests related to my sporting injury were carried out by a sports injury specialist.

This was my last meeting with my original GP who missed the original signs of my blood disease.

My heart attack occurred after my new GP referred me to a heart clinic with chest pain.

At the clinic on the same day, I performed a stress test on the treadmill while I was hooked up to an ECG (electrocardiogram) machine, and I only lasted approximately two minutes before acute chest pains forced me to stop the test.

I was greatly concerned by these events and explained to the heart specialist that this was a dramatic and severe reduction in function, as I was an ex-triathlete and long-distance runner normally able to complete these tests easily.

He agreed that something was wrong and scheduled me for an exploratory angiogram in six weeks' time.

I expressed my concern over this timetable but again, I did not appear sick, or in imminent danger on the outside, but I knew that my heart function and ability to exercise had been dramatically and quickly reduced.

I went home and four days later, had a heart attack while mowing the lawn.

While having my heart attack I was able to call my GP, who coordinated the arrangements at the private hospital emergency department while we waited for the ambulance to arrive.

They arrived in about seven minutes, entering the house and taking my blood pressure immediately.

They advised that my blood pressure was about 220 over 180 and I was indeed having a heart attack.

The next question threw me and provided another opportunity for a dad joke when the paramedics asked if me if I had taken Viagra in the last hour.

I said, "I am fucked, not fucking, why would you ask me that?"

They loved my answer, and after a quick laugh advised that Viagra could interact with the medication (Nitrolingual – glyceryl trinitrate) they were about to administer to relieve the heart attack symptoms and lower the blood pressure too far.

Upon admission at the hospital, as it was a Saturday the heart surgeon and his team had to be called in. In the cardiac centre, my first words to the heart surgeon were, "I told you that my heart was worse that you thought, and I nearly died waiting for the test. Six weeks was too long."

I was not in a position of strength at the time, as he was about to shove a tube up through my femoral artery into my heart to insert a stent, so I chose to drop it after that and be nice while the procedure continued.

You remain awake through this procedure, so I lay back and watched it all happen.

I might add that the heart surgeon has my full support and has been a caring professional who has produced a spectacular outcome for me. I remain in his care and he has my full respect for his technical knowledge and the application of his knowledge.

My only point of contention remains that the medical system is generally overloaded, so waiting to see specialists or to have certain surgical procedures and/or tests can be weeks or months, even with private healthcare. Sometimes, the wait can be a genuine risk to your health.

The diagnosis with the bilateral clear cell renal carcinomas (CCRC) in both kidneys was another example of right over might.

I had been to a long business lunch and had a great day consuming many alcoholic beverages (mainly beer).

Later in the night I started vomiting profusely and violently and had searing pain down both sides of my abdomen in what felt like my kidneys.

I had vomited in my life before, but had never experienced pain of this magnitude, so we went immediately to the emergency department of the nearest hospital, a public hospital.

I advised the triage nurse of the severity of my symptoms and was in so much pain the only relief I could get was lying on the floor of the emergency room.

They quickly moved me into the emergency assessment room and administered a large dose of intravenous pain medication.

This hardly worked, and I remained in a lot of pain, which concerned the medical staff (and me).

I had chest x-rays, blood tests and more pain medication and during this period I continually said that the pain was in my kidneys.

The medical staff kept assuring me that kidney pain does not present in the manner I was describing, and I kept arguing with them that the pain was in my kidneys and I wanted my kidneys examined.

This ridiculous argument continued for over 12 hours, where I met with a new shift of doctors and nurses and had the same argument, maintaining that they needed to check my kidneys, and them saying that I had a virus or a hangover or both, but the pain was not emanating from my kidneys.

By 4 o'clock the next day, I was still in pain in the emergency assessment room arguing about a scan being conducted on my kidneys. I told them that I had presented to the emergency ward with pain in my kidneys, I still had the pain in my kidneys and they had tested every bloody thing except my kidneys, so unless they agreed to conduct some tests on my kidneys I would be leaving and seeking admission to another hospital and lodging a formal complaint against them for failing to deal with the issue.

The doctor eventually reluctantly agreed to an ultrasound scan of my kidneys. Only two minutes into the ultrasound, the technician apologised and left the room for approximately half an hour, while I just lay there.

When she returned, the mood had turned sombre and there was no further discussion apart from her advice that she had had to consult with a specialist, and they would meet with me after the scan.

When I returned to the bed in the emergency assessment room, I was the only patient left in there. The whole medical team was gathered around a computer and looking very worried and then looking back at me.

I said to my wife that unfortunately it appeared I was right about the kidneys and the news would be bad.

This observation was too close to the truth, as after about 20 minutes the head medical doctor came over and sat down by the bed and advised us that they had discovered tumours on both kidneys.

The tumour on the right kidney was approximately four centimetres in diameter and the one on the left one to two centimetres.

So, I had a stage 4 CCRC on my right kidney and a stage 2 CCRC on my left.

He said that if left unchecked, the tumours would have progressed until the symptoms such as blood in the urine appeared and by then, my life expectancy would be very low and removal of both kidneys and dialysis treatment was a certainty.

He advised that I was likely to have the right kidney surgically removed and possibly be placed on dialysis with my current diagnosis, but he would arrange an appointment with a specialist as soon as possible to discuss the options.

I thanked him for his professionalism and compassion, but I also reminded him that I had presented with bilateral abdominal pain which I was adamant emanated from my kidneys and had wanted my kidneys tested.

The doctors apologised to me and explained that normally, CCRC does not occur in both kidneys (I cover this later in the book, but less than 2% of the population contracts CCRC in both kidneys), and also pain such as I described was not normally associated with the kidneys.

I know that a patient must rely on the knowledge and experience of the doctors, but sometimes they must also listen to the patient.

If they had scanned my kidneys when I first presented at the hospital and found nothing, then they could have moved to the next possible cause if they were correct in their diagnosis.

If they had listened to me and scanned the kidneys first,

I would not have been in hospital under emergency care for almost 24 hours. I would not have had the x-rays and blood tests which came back inconclusive, I would have had better pain management and they would have discovered the condition much earlier.

Tip Number 4

Sometimes medical treatment comes at a cost, but sometimes the cost determines the treatment.

Tip Number 5

Once you get a serious diagnosis, start straightaway on improving your overall health and fitness through diet, exercise and relaxation activities, consistent with your individual personal circumstances and medical condition.

Your GP should be able to assist with general advice on these activities before you commence a new or improved exercise and diet regime.

From my discussions with various medical practitioners while researching this book, their collective assessments of patients faced with a dire cancer diagnosis show that only approximately 5–10% of patients embark on a healthy regime to be as fit and healthy as possible before commencing treatment.

A lot of patients merely accept the diagnosis and give themselves over to the treatment and the associated outcomes.

In my view, this fatalistic approach is not utilising the available healing functions of the body to its full potential.

Chapter 2

Diagnosis Confirmation, Dealing with Tests, Preparing for Treatment

Quite often, once a serious medical condition such as cancer is diagnosed, further scans and tests are required to establish the location and/or spread of the disease, if tumours are present and whether it is a primary or secondary cancer.

These tests may also be required to assess the treatment options, such as whether surgery and excision, or chemo-therapy and/or radiation or other treatment options should be considered. They can be confronting and it takes resilience and application to complete them.

It is not possible to cover the scope of all cancers and medical conditions in this book. The necessary tests and procedures to confirm a diagnosis or formulate a treatment regime differ greatly with each individual and their particular condition/s.

The advice in this book is based on my experiences, generally covering the basic type of scans, tests and procedures that cancer patients may face and how to prepare for this phase of the treatment.

Some of the most common forms of cancer treatment are:

Surgery
Removal of cancer from your body by a surgeon.

Radiation therapy or x-ray therapy
X-rays destroy or impede the growth of cancer cells or relieve pain associated with incurable diseases. Radiotherapy can also be utilised in conjunction with other cancer treatments.

Chemotherapy
The use of drugs which can destroy or impede the growth of cancer cells. Chemotherapy treatments can consist of one or more drugs depending upon the cancer being treated.

Immunotherapy
This treatment focuses on the use of the patient's own immune system to fight and attack the cancer by boosting the immune system, slow the rate of growth of the cancer and remove the barriers to the immune system attacking the cancer.

Targeted therapy
(biological therapy, and molecular targeted therapy)
The use of specialised drug treatments that identify and attack cancer cells aimed at stopping the growth and spread of cancer in the patient.

Hormone therapy
Most commonly used for the treatment of prostate, uterine and breast cancer and involves the removal of the hormone-producing glands to stop the spread and growth of cancer cells.

Stem cell transplant or bone marrow transplant
Used for the treatment of blood cancers such as lymphoma, leukaemia or myeloma and involves the replacement of blood-forming cells in your body, such as cancer cells or cells which have been adversely affected by radiation or chemotherapy treatment, with new healthy stem cells which grow into new bone marrow and healthy blood cells. These transplants can use your own stem cells (autologous transplant) or donor stem cells (allogenic transplant). The stem cell collection process is arduous, and my experiences with this process are detailed later in this book.

Precision or personalised medicine
Involves the use of genomics and a greater knowledge of the patient's DNA to provide tailored disease prevention

and treatment using the patient's own genes, environment and lifestyle. The concept applies the analysis of a patient's genetic makeup to construct and target treatments based on the specific needs of the individual.

Some of the tests that you may face include, but are not limited to, those listed below.

Magnetic Resonance Imaging (MRI) used to form pictures of the anatomy and the physiological processes of the body using strong magnetic fields.

Computerised tomography (CT scan) is a combination of x-rays taken from different angles around the body. A CT scan can then use computer processing to compile cross-sectional images of skeletal structures, blood vessels and soft tissue with a much more detailed result than x-rays.

Positron Emission Tomography, better known as PET scans, are used to detect small tumours by obtaining images of the cells of the body while they are working. These scans use a special dye with radioactive elements that are traced by the equipment. The radioactive tracers are usually injected, swallowed or inhaled by the patient prior to the scan commencing.

Usually a scan requires the patient to lie prone and enter the scanning equipment. The time taken varies with the type of scan and tests being undertaken and some patients suffer from the fear of confined spaces.

I have had spinal taps, where fluid is taken from the spine for analysis, too many blood samples taken to count and kidney biopsies and other treatments associated with my particular circumstances. Regardless of the test or scan to be performed, some basic issues remain constant, including:

- The tests are generally required to maximise your information and assist the treating medical practitioners
- Most of these procedures involve discomfort of some sort, so research the procedure and plan your attendance and participation to suit the requirements.

Find out when the results of the procedure will be available and sent to your doctor so that you can arrange an appointment to discuss the results.

Use relaxation techniques to get through the procedure and focus on positive thoughts and how the information will be used, rather than on the discomfort of the procedure.

Remember that this is just part of the process.

Tip Number 6

If you are unsure of the need for a particular expensive or invasive test or procedure, raise it with your treating doctor and ask why it is necessary and if there are other options.

Blood tests will generally be required to assess general health and define abnormalities associated with your condition.

Where patients are about to undergo chemotherapy and/or numerous blood tests or infusions, they are generally offered the choice of having a portacath or central line inserted into their body just under the skin, close to the heart.

A portacath or a central line allows chemotherapy and other drugs and fluids to be delivered without the need for an injection.

A portacath can stay in place for two to six years (if required). It sits under the skin and cannot be seen, whereas a central line has a tube coming out of your chest.

Patients who don't like having needles every time they need treatment prefer either a portacath or central line.

A central line also allows blood to be drawn as required without needles.

There can be complications from infection, blood clots or blockages with these apparatuses, and if you are not having regular treatment the apparatus will need to be cleaned and flushed by a nurse.

In my case I decided not to have a portacath or central line for the following reasons:

- It would be a constant reminder that I was undergoing chemotherapy and had cancer

- I did not want any physical restrictions while not undergoing treatment
- I was concerned about the risks of infection and the maintenance of the apparatus
- I was not concerned about needles
- I had reasonably accessible veins.

There are obviously risks and rewards with each option. As with other parts of this book, I can only relate to you my personal experiences and how I dealt with them during my treatment so that you are aware of some of the issues you may face, and how to make the decisions that provide the best outcome for you.

The biggest downside I discovered by not having the portacath or central line was that each time I had blood taken or had an intravenous line inserted for an infusion, I had to rely on the expertise of the person inserting the needle or line at the time.

The level of expertise varied from totally incompetent to blissfully professional.

On many occasions the nurse inserting the needle failed to locate the vein and took many attempts to find a suitable placement.

Due to the damage caused to veins by so many needle insertions over the course of my treatment, I would use one arm only (I was saving the other arm for next time if I needed it).

I would tell the nurses where the vein was and provide advice on what the past successful nurse had done to get the best outcome.

Some nurses just tried a few times on one arm and wanted to try the other arm and occasionally I would agree, but most times I told them to calm down, take a break and try again or get someone who knew how to do it properly.

There is nothing worse than being about to commence an infusion of chemotherapy drugs and being poked and stabbed with a needle, and the nurse saying things like, "I can't find a vein, this is not working today."

On a couple of occasions, I told the nurses to get someone else, as I was not prepared to sit through any more practice for them.

This procedure requires patience, practice and pro-fessionalism. One nurse who took the blood samples while I was in hospital for my stem cell collection process was so proficient that each time he collected blood from me it was painless, quick and accurate.

That proved to me that it is only the level of competence that varies, not the patient's veins or other excuses used when you are sitting there bleeding from unsuccessful puncture wounds with the nurse unable to find a vein.

This is one drawback of not having the portacath, but if

faced with the same choices, I would do the same again and opt for the needles rather than the permanent portacath or central line.

It is common for nurses or doctors to recommend a portacath or central line prior to commencing your treatment. At least after reading about my experiences, you'll be in a position to discuss your concerns with the treating doctor to arrive at the best possible option for you.

If you choose not to have the portacath or central line, but then find that the needles are causing too many problems, it is relatively easy to reverse your decision and have an apparatus inserted.

I endured many varied tests prior to the commencement of my treatment and despite the best efforts of the medical practitioners involved, occasionally things did not go as planned. You must be ready to deal with these aberrations, as the tests must be completed.

During one spinal tap or lumbar puncture, the practitioner failed six times to insert the needle into my spine correctly. A spinal tap is required to remove a sample of cerebrospinal fluid from between two lumbar bones. A local anaesthetic to the lower back or spine is first applied, then a needle is inserted between the vertebrae and the fluid is collected for analysis.

Regardless of the local anaesthetic, the pain and discomfort were intense. I was unable to do anything about the situation, so I chose to meditate and went back to a recent triathlon I had raced in, running the race again in my head with my eyes closed.

When the practitioner kept apologising for his inability to insert the needle, I told him that I was meditating and not to talk to me, just to get the job done.

I also reminded him that at some stage, the procedure would be finished and I would be getting up off the table. I strongly believed in sharing my experience equally, so the more pain he inflicted on me the higher the chances that I would reciprocate on him when I got up.

He laughed at these comments, which were heard by others in the region (he had asked for assistance when the procedure was not going well, and my wife and other patients were within hearing distance), but it appeared to work as he got the needle in pretty much straight after our discussion.

In today's world of political correctness these comments could have been construed as threatening, but they were not meant or taken that way. They were a way of easing the tension of a very uncomfortable situation for all of us.

You will find throughout this book examples of comments or behaviours made by me or others that may appear to be confrontational or inappropriate. My view is that at the time they were entirely appropriate, and I have lived to tell the tale.

Tip Number 7

If it hurts, it's not working or you are uncomfortable, tell somebody, stick up for yourself, ask questions, seek other opinions, get somebody who knows how to do the procedure. Don't suffer in silence and hope that things will improve on their own.

Always be polite and respectful but firm, and don't forget humour can diffuse many difficult situations.

Before any test, prepare yourself by considering the following points:

1. Understand the test, the need for the test and the conditions of the test, e.g. fasting and liquids allowed before and after the test.
2. What are the possible side effects of any drugs, radiation or activity associated with the test.
3. What are the costs of the test, and any possible rebates or concessions you may be able to claim.
4. Make sure you know the location of the test/procedure, and allow enough time to arrive, find a parking space or disembark from public transport and calm down before commencing the process.
5. If you meditate, listen to music or a relaxation podcast or app on your phone or tablet while waiting.

6. Recognise that you are the most important person in your life, but to the testing staff and facility you are patient number x and one of possibly hundreds who will go through their facility on the day of your test. Things will not always go as planned, so roll with the punches and stay positive.

7. Even if the test procedure is cancelled, it will be rescheduled.

8. Remember that the test or procedure is the start of your treatment process and a step closer to battling the cancer.

9. Have a family member or support person with you if possible, and if not, make arrangements to get transport home as you may be unable to drive or be mobile.

10. Even if fasting is not a requirement, be practical with your activities and diet prior to the test. A big night out on the booze followed by a big breakfast and a couple of cups of coffee is not the best way to prepare for some of these procedures, and may hinder your ability to tolerate chemicals, drugs and certain activities.

After the tests have been completed, it is essential to discuss the results with your treating medical practitioners in a manner that you can comprehend and in jargon that you can understand.

If you are being 'blinded by science' and terminology that is unfamiliar to you, request a layman's explanation of the terms.

It is usually after all the tests and scans have been completed that the decisions on the type of treatment and the options you as the patient need to consider are discussed.

These decisions can be life altering and need careful consideration, so don't be forced into making on-the-spot decisions. If you have concerns, ask for more time and another appointment if possible.

Women are often faced with choices such as the removal of breasts through single or double mastectomies, or in other cases the removal of their reproductive organs through hysterectomies.

These decisions and outcomes have significant personal and psychological impacts on the patient and their futures. They need very careful consideration, in conjunction with competent medical advice, before irreversible decisions of this nature are made.

Men also face complex decisions in relation to prostate cancer where their options may be watch and wait, or surgery with risks such as incontinence and impotency. Complex decisions apply to most cancers and decisions that must be made.

Research is key, and while you must rely on the quali-fications and experience of the treating medical practitioners, you are the one who has to live with the consequences of your choices and decisions associated with your illness and your treatment.

Tip Number 8

Have faith in your doctor/specialist and if you don't, seek another opinion and/or referral.

Chapter 3

Questions to ask your GP and Treating Specialist/s Before Treatment

Before commencing any treatment, in my case high doses of chemotherapy drugs and surgery, I found it helpful to start a notebook which recorded my weight, blood pressure, cholesterol, BMI, waist measurement, glucose reading and whatever other baseline results obtained from the tests, scans, etc.

This notebook was a great reference point for me after a few months of treatment because I could compare my before and after treatment details.

I also logged entries detailing my exercise before and after treatment, and how I felt after each chemotherapy treatment and following exercise sessions.

Many of the side effects and associated impacts of the

treatment were not explained to me before the treatment in detail, although I was advised that usually day eight or nine after a chemotherapy infusion was the worst day when I would feel the sickest.

Again, I must state that my treating medical practitioners and nurses were professional and gave me as much information as they could at the time, but as they have never actually taken the drugs themselves it is difficult for them to relate to some of the associated side effects.

Indeed, before commencing my chemotherapy treatment, the treating oncologist at the private health facility arranged a meeting with me and my family to discuss the upcoming treatment and some of the things that I could expect during the course of chemotherapy drugs.

This was a morose and very formal discussion, and although technically well delivered, everybody in the room looked sad and members of my family shed a few tears.

My prognosis at that time was not great, as I had been advised that if the treatment was unsuccessful I would probably have less than six months to live.

When we were going through the possible side effects of the chemotherapy drugs, the doctor asked me if I had any questions. I said that I did, and this is how the conversation went.

Doctor: Do you have any questions?

Me: Yes, can I still play tennis during the treatment?

Doctor: Yes, if you feel up to it, as it depends on the individual and how they react to the chemotherapy drugs.

Me: Can I still go for a run?

Doctor: Yes, if you feel up to it, as it depends on the individual and how they react to the chemotherapy drugs.

Me: Can I have sex during the treatment?

Doctor: Not recommended, as the chemotherapy drugs may be passed to your partner through the body fluids. (Wow, this was news to me!) Also, libido is significantly reduced by the chemotherapy drugs.

Me: Can I play the piano?

Doctor: Yes, you can if you feel up to it, as it depends on the individual and how they react to the chemotherapy drugs.

Me: That's great, because I have never been able to play the piano before.

This ill-timed dad joke cracked me up but got little recognition or applause from my audience at the time.

To this day I can still see all their faces after the punchline and it cheers me up.

Tip Number 9

Try and find something funny in almost everything you do. Believe me, it helps.

The more you feel sad and sorry for yourself, the more this feeling will be reflected in others.

If you are facing surgery or radiation treatment or some other form of intervention, most of the preparation points remain the same as outlined in Chapter 2 of this book.

The process can be treated as a race like a triathlon or marathon where preparation, fitness and attitude greatly influence the outcome.

Chemotherapy infusions can be particularly daunting as you are faced with sessions of from four hours to six or seven hours depending on the treatment, the location and many other factors.

Most of my treatments lasted for four to five hours and believe me, the first one is daunting.

To go from your everyday comfort zone to a medical facility, have a needle placed into your arm/wrist, and then be hooked up to chemicals that you know will make you ill at some stage is confronting to anyone.

I dealt with it by being prepared, which started by shaving off my thick dark hair.

This act invoked its own tale, as I went to my local shopping centre, walked into the nearest hairdresser's and asked the hairdresser to shave my head.

I was dressed in business clothes, looked in reasonable health and had a full head of dark hair.

Her response was that a head shave was a very dramatic act, and she was unwilling to do so, as some customers who had had such radical haircuts and changes in appearance had occasionally taken their frustrations out on the hairdresser.

While I could understand her point of view, I explained that I had recently been diagnosed with stage 4 non-Hodgkin lymphoma and was about to undergo chemotherapy treatment which would result in total hair loss.

I got the haircut I requested and her sympathy, but you will find that telling complete strangers about your condition is harder than it sounds, and I tried to limit these discussions where possible.

In hindsight, my decision suited my circumstances at the time, and I owned the bald look.

When I was asked by friends and acquaintances why I had shaved my head, I merely responded with 'trying out a new streamlined look' and this usually worked.

For people who knew of my diagnosis and treatment, the new look became a point of fun and I laughed along with it.

Having a swim/surf/shower became easier and still after

11 years I wear my hair short (number 2 buzz cut) and have embraced the look.

At one stage of the treatment there was not a single hair on my body, and this was confronting, but in my view the chemicals that killed the hair were also killing the cancer cells, so in my mind the lack of hair was a sign that the treatment was working.

On one occasion, approximately two years after the chemotherapy ceased, I had a stem cell collection which involved a day-long infusion of chemotherapy chemicals and some serious side effects which I will go into later in this book.

During this process I decided to leave my hair intact (it had grown back by then) and see what happened.

This proved to be a bad decision, as each time I showered or brushed my hair it came out in clumps and left patchy holes on my scalp.

It also reminded me constantly that I was unwell and having serious treatment to save my life, so I shaved it off again.

Another interesting phenomenon is that quite often when the hair regrows after chemotherapy, on both men and women the new hair that comes back is a different colour, crinkly and curly and much resembling pubic hair.

Again, my remedy was to shave my head a few more times and eventually it straightened out.

I realise that some patients, particularly women, may suffer more than men over the loss of hair. Again, my advice is to plan for it by consulting cancer support groups before the treatment and hair loss, and explore options including cosmetic treatments, hats, bandanas and wigs.

One of the recent innovations in this area is the use of a cancer cooling cap or scalp cooling systems.

These caps are a tightly fitting, strap-on helmet type of hat that is filled with a gel coolant chilled to between -26 to -40 degrees Celsius (-15 to -40 degrees Fahrenheit).

The purpose of the cooling caps is to narrow the blood vessels underneath the skin of the scalp, which in turn reduces the amount of chemotherapy medicines that reach the hair follicles of the patient.

This reduces the likelihood of the hair falling out. The low temperature also reduces the activity of the hair follicles which can lessen the impact of the chemotherapy medicine on them.

The cooling caps are worn for 20–50 minutes before the treatment commences, as well as during and after the treatment.

Once again, the efficacy of a cooling cap is relative to your condition and the type of cancer being treated, and their use would depend upon your chemotherapy regime and any other health issues applicable to your case.

Current research shows that these caps have been found to be effective in about 50–65% of patients.

The cooling caps are not free. They can be purchased for between $1,500 and $3,000 and are generally not covered by health insurance.

Feeling good about yourself is important and there are many ways to deal with hair loss and appearance changes.

In my view, staying at home, in hospital or out of the general population only increases anxiety and limits your recovery.

On my first day of treatment I had a family member with me (my wife) and either a family member or friend for each treatment after that.

I took magazines and my laptop, and had relaxation music and comedy podcasts loaded onto my iPod as well as my mobile phone.

I had no idea what to expect, and once I sat in the high-backed chair and had the infusion line inserted into my arm with a saline drip to get things started, I realised that this was serious. I had to keep my thoughts positive or the whole process would become a nightmare.

I quickly realised that anxiety and depression could ruin the experience and hinder my recovery, so on that first day I set goals to stay positive, keep what I could control under control and let the doctors and the medicine do their job.

This does not mean that everything was unicorns and

flowers. On the contrary, things were quite dire, but I tried to manage my thoughts to accept on the one hand that I had been diagnosed with a serious and life-threatening illness, and on the other, that I needed to try and maximise my attributes and not be dragged down by negativity.

Once I was hooked up to the machine and could feel the drugs entering my system, I concentrated on holding a discussion with my support person, reading or working on my laptop.

There is no doubt that it is a daunting feeling to actually be aware of the drugs going into your veins, and some of the drugs cause an instant reaction.

One of the drugs that was included in my chemotherapy treatment was vincristine, which is so toxic that the nurses placed ice cubes inside my mouth while the drug was being administered and warned me that I would feel a sensation that my body was heating up from the inside.

This was good advice, but my description after the event would be more along the lines of comparing it to the feeling you would get if you swallowed a cup of sulphuric acid.

Thankfully, the feeling did not last long.

Next time, I was prepared for it and was not as alarmed by the symptoms.

The symptoms described below associated with vin-cristine will give you some idea of what I went through, bearing in mind that I had no idea that these side effects were associated with this drug at the time.

Common side effects of vincristine sulfate injection include nausea, vomiting, weight loss, diarrhoea, bloating, stomach/abdominal pain or cramps, mouth sores, dizziness, headache, hair loss, constipation, loss of appetite, changes in sense of taste and numbness and tingling in the hands and feet.

Hence my advice to research these drugs if possible and discuss the possible side effects with your doctor before commencing the treatment.

Having the information about the side effects at the time would not have changed my need for the drug, but knowing what to expect would have made the process less confronting.

At the time, I owned and operated a human resources, industrial relations, mediation and dispute settlement consulting company which was very successful and my principal source of income.

Throughout my treatments I continued to work, simply because I needed a distraction from the medical roundabout I was on, and it gave me focus and mental stimulation.

Once I became used to the infusion process, I would get up (while still hooked up to the chemicals) and go for a walk on the floor of the treatment room to the toilet, or chat with another patient, leaving my support person who was also well prepared to read a book or use their own electronic devices.

I cannot stress how important it is to have a family member or support person with you if at all possible through these treatments, as their presence is calming and reassuring.

If you are in a position where this is not possible, try and find another patient who has no family or support person and talk to them. They will appreciate your company, and if not, they will generally let you know.

Once I discovered that I felt reasonably well immediately after the chemotherapy infusion session, I turned the occasion into a celebration, and whoever came with me got shouted to a late lunch at the Sheraton Hotel on the waterfront on the Gold Coast, which was not far from the treatment facility.

Decisions about the efficacy of the treatment and your progress are best left to the medical specialists and discussed throughout the process. However, some decisions although difficult can be made by you so that you are in charge of your own destiny.

On one occasion approximately five days after my third chemotherapy infusion, I was very ill. I remember looking in the bathroom mirror and seeing my image. I had lost approximately 10 kilos, I did not have a hair on my body, my skin was white and almost translucent, I had no energy, I felt nauseated and generally as low as I could go.

About an hour after this event, I was contacted by my

haematologist who advised me that after my latest blood test my red blood cell count was dangerously low (around 60; a healthy reading is around 150). He advised that if the blood count dropped below 60 there was a real chance that I would die, and it was likely that I would need to go to hospital quickly and have a full blood transfusion.

I had total faith in his medical competence and management of my illness, but I also considered my position concerning this latest development and the following points.

1. A full blood transfusion would remove all of the chemotherapy drugs that were in my system, specifically from the most recent infusion.
2. The blood would have to come from someone else's body.
3. It might fix the problem of the low blood count, but the cancer would get a free kick.
4. This would prolong the chemotherapy treatments and possibly exacerbate the side effects.
5. I was immune compromised, very weak and losing resilience and another medical procedure was not at the top of my list.

While in such a weakened state I considered the options and advised the doctor that I would not have the transfusion. I would take my chances that the chemotherapy treatments to date would kick in and destroy the mutated blood cancer cells and new ones would start to grow.

I will just say that this was a tough decision, and I realised that I could actually die from the disease if my blood count continued to decline and my anaemia grew unchecked.

I took the steps to advise my wife and two adult children that I had made this decision and was fully aware of the consequences.

I also advised them that this was serious, and that it was quite possible I would be dead within months unless there was significant improvement.

While this was a difficult conversation and decision, I was at the time clear that it was the best of my options. After looking in the mirror earlier in the day, it looked like I was well on the way to the end of my life.

I felt quite calm after this decision was made, and just carried on normally as best I could for a few days, not sure what my longevity might be.

About four days later, I noticed some pink colouration in my fingernails which had not been there a few days before.

I notified my doctor, and we arranged another blood test to measure my haemoglobin count.

The results were encouraging with the count now around 76, so things appeared to be improving.

Based on this improvement in my red blood cell count, I continued with the remaining chemotherapy treatments.

Each one delivered its own challenges, but I became used to the routine and just stuck my arm out ready for the needle.

This decision was one of many I made on my journey. Some may not agree with them, but they were the right decisions for me at the time and they worked for me.

One of my most radical decisions was to continue running while undergoing the chemotherapy treatment.

My view was that my particular cancer was in my bone marrow and circulatory system, and just lying around feeling sorry for myself after chemotherapy treatments was not going to achieve much.

I figured that for the chemicals to get all around my body and into my bone marrow they needed to be shaken up a bit.

My greatest asset was that prior to the diagnosis I had been super fit, had a well-balanced diet and had not consumed alcohol or eaten red meat for approximately 17 years.

My GP at one stage commented that I was not as fit as an elite athlete, I was in fact an elite athlete.

I was an accomplished long-distance runner, triathlete, tennis player and pretty much a fitness fanatic, and in great shape for my age of 55 when diagnosed.

My dedication to training and my pain management techniques greatly assisted me through my illness and its various treatments.

Just prior to being diagnosed, I competed in the team that

won the longest running race in the Southern Hemisphere (the then named Endeavour 500), a 500-kilometre foot race completed over a three-day period.

I trained with the team and on my own all year for four or five years while we competed in this annual event, and it became my motivation and life goal outside my family and work interests.

Sometimes when undergoing treatment, I would close my eyes and think that if I could run over Cunningham's Gap at the top of the Great Dividing Range in Queensland against runners of the calibre of Pat Carrol (Australian Marathon Champion) and Andrew Lloyd (Commonwealth Games Gold Medal runner) in around 40 degree heat, then I should be able to tolerate suffering some discomfort during a chemotherapy treatment.

I know that everybody is different and each person must use the tools they have to deal with this journey. I am just recounting how I dealt with it so you have some understanding of the fact that undergoing these treatments is a holistic process that requires application, dedication, trust and some good luck.

Chapter 4

Going Through Treatment

Cancer treatment, no matter the type or location of the cancer, is usually a serious and complex matter with decisions to be made by many people and institutions.

The patient generally has to leave their relatively comfortable life bubble and enter a new world made up of a many-faceted health system involving bureaucracy, medical practices, testing organisations, other patients, drugs, equipment and people.

This system has the ability to perform its required functions, but to do so well it requires coordination, expertise, knowledge, IT, administration systems and in most cases, money.

As a patient, you need to be prepared for entering this system.

As a newly diagnosed cancer patient about to commence treatment, I found that uncertainty and the inability to control the chain of events unfolding was causing me some distress. I was determined to rein in these feelings in order to concentrate all of my efforts on getting through the treatment and achieving the best outcome possible.

To help with this process, I performed tasks that removed uncertainty and made my life easier.

The first thing I did was to get my affairs in order. This included organising an update of my will, making an enduring power of attorney and an advance health directive (which detailed my wishes in case I was incapable of making decisions), organising my work and advising clients.

My advance health directive gave me reassurance that if things did go bad, my decisions about medication, treatment and resuscitation would be clearly defined and honoured by the treating medical staff and my family.

I also recorded all my passwords and banking and finance details in a book that could be easily accessed by my wife.

I made sure that my private healthcare provider payments were paid monthly by deduction from my bank account, and that the account had sufficient funds at all times to cover this payment.

Although to some people this may seem a negative step, in my view the knowledge that I had these processes and documents in place gave me a few less things to worry about.

Once the treatment is ready to commence, most hospital

admissions for surgery and/or radiation treatment can be frustrating and long.

It is general practice that once the surgeon has scheduled the surgery/procedure and all the tests and admission papers are completed, you are required to attend the hospital usually around 5.30 to 6 am.

The procedures described below are based on my personal experiences with surgery over the last 10 to 12 years.

The first step before a surgery commences is the initial check-in at the hospital and then a wait in the general waiting room. Then you move to the first surgical waiting room where your details are confirmed, the procedure discussed and you change into a hospital gown and dressing gown and slippers.

After that, you go into a second separate surgical waiting room to wait for your scheduled procedure.

By this time your glasses, watch, phone and any contact with the outside world have been removed and you are in a roomful of strangers watching breakfast television on a centrally located TV.

Depending upon where you are on the list, you may be there for a few hours, and if complications occur and you are not the first patient in the operating theatre it may be a long wait.

I take in with me an old book that I don't care if I lose. Generally, the nurses will let you take something in with you.

I also take to the hospital an old watch and a small amount of cash in an old wallet with only my healthcare cards.

There is no guarantee that your phone will make it back to your room if you take it with you. It can be risky.

I used the waiting time before surgery to positively reflect on why I was there and what the positive benefits of the process were. I started to plan my recovery strategy and visualised running along the beach with the cancer removed and a few scars to show what had occurred.

Most people have some apprehension before undergoing major invasive surgery. The whole process can be quite intimidating, particularly when you are wheeled through the doors into the main operating theatre.

There are a lot of large bright lights, people dressed in surgical gowns and masks and a lot of scary looking equipment.

In my case for my most recent surgery there were large robotic arms all covered in plastic which contributed to the scary scene.

In my last surgery, I had had an initial injection to relax me and was feeling mellow and ready to go, when the surgeon came in and said he had some bad news for me.

Get that picture in your mind. I arrived at the hospital at 5.30 am as requested, went through all the required procedures, waited in the waiting area for about 90 minutes, was given a pre-op injection, and was waiting to go through the doors and commence the operation when my surgeon said he had bad news.

The news he delivered was that the machine that monitored my kidney function during the surgery (partial nephrectomy to remove a stage 4 CCRC from the kidney) was double booked. They suggested that I go back to the waiting room and instead of being the first to be operated on (I was first on the list due to the complexity of my surgery), they would commence the operation at approximately 4.30 pm instead of 8.30 am as scheduled.

I said that it was unacceptable, that the circumstances had placed me in a very difficult position, that I was booked for the surgery, already prepped and ready to go. I asked to see the person who had made the fuck-up with the bookings and said I would be seeking to have that person sacked. I would consider legal action against them and the hospital for this distressing set of circumstances.

I was not prepared to return to the waiting room for another 8–10 hours, or for the possibility that the surgery was postponed if the other surgeries on the list went longer than expected or had complications, just because some administration clerk had failed to do their job.

My surgery had been booked for weeks and this failure should not have occurred.

It was clear that I was becoming quite agitated and distressed and my blood pressure was going through the roof. I reminded the surgeon that I had had a recent heart attack and this was giving me chest pains and anxiety. I said that he needed to fix this issue as I was very unhappy at the bad news.

He went away and returned about 10 minutes later saying that the surgery would proceed as planned. I asked if the required machine was available for my surgery because I was not going to risk my life because the machine was not available.

I was advised that the required machine had been secured for my surgery and it would proceed as planned.

Great start to serious surgery. This is not how one should enter an operating theatre.

I used meditation and breathing techniques to lower my blood pressure quickly and I was wheeled in.

As soon as I was on the operating table, the anaesthetist commandeered my arm and was preparing to administer the knock-out drugs. I knew that I only had a few seconds and I couldn't resist the moment, so I yelled, "Dr … told me that if this surgery goes well, you'll all get a $10,000 bonus!" Then I was out like a light.

I must add that at all times the surgeon was caring and professional and his technical skills saved my kidney and prolonged my life. His handling of the issue was exemplary.

I generally treat going under anaesthetic for surgery as a positive experience, and in my mind, it is as close as possible to time travel. All you have to do is turn up and be calm. Once you are under the anaesthetic, everything you have control over stops. You then wake up some hours later in a surgical ward with the surgery completed and full of nice drugs.

How good is that!

If for some reason you do not wake up, then you won't know anything about it anyway, so either way there will be a result.

Tip Number 10

Dignity, status and modesty quickly become casualties of testing, treatment and hospitalisation.

Don't worry about walking around a hospital with your gown undone down the back and your bum hanging out. Believe me, no one cares. It's the same for everyone, just part of hospital life.

Your appearance and dress while undergoing some of these procedures and treatments is the last thing you should worry about.

There are over one million people employed in the delivery of health and welfare services in Australia, over 150 million healthcare workers in America and 1.9 million in England at the time of writing this book.

When you enter the system, you practically become a number to be treated, tracked and billed. While in general this will be carried out efficiently and with care, the propensity for errors and actions that can cause issues, from irritability and discomfort to death, are real and must be identified and managed so that as a patient you receive the best care and outcomes possible.

There are conflicting views and reports available in Australia regarding claims that private hospitals have smaller nurse-to-patient ratios than public hospitals.

While this may be a factor to consider, the private hospitals generally have better conditions, your own choice of doctor and a shorter surgical waiting list.

This is too big a subject to cover in this book. However, it has been my experience that during my stays in both private and public hospitals, there is a noticeable lack of nursing staff in the private hospitals, particularly on night shift and at weekends when labour costs are at their highest.

Figures available at the time of writing found that in Australia, 7.7 % of surgical admissions and 4.7% of non -surgical admissions experienced an adverse event.

The following is an extract from the Australian Commission on Safety and Quality in Health Care 2019

Report, *The State of Patient Safety and Quality in Australian Hospitals 2019:*[*]

> The personal and financial impact of patient safety lapses is considerable. In 2013, approximately 12% to 16.5% of total hospital activity and expenditure was the direct result of adverse events. In the financial year 2017–18, admissions associated with hospital-acquired complications (HACs)[†] were estimated by the Australian Commission on Safety and Quality in Health Care (the Commission) to cost the public sector $4.1 billion[‡] or 8.9%[§] of total hospital expenditure. The most burdensome adverse event types include healthcare-associated infections (HAIs), medication complications, delirium and cardiac complications.

In America, a median of 10% of patients was affected by an adverse event, with a median of 7.3% being fatal and between 34.3% and 83% being preventable (BMC Health Services research published online 4 July 2018 https://www.ncbi.nlm.nih.gov/pmc/articles/PMC6032777/).

In England, 10.8% of patients experienced an adverse event, with one third of adverse events leading to moderate or greater disability or death (PubMedCentral https://www.ncbi.nlm.nih.gov/pmc/articles/PMC26554/).

---

[*]   https://www.safetyandquality.gov.au/publications-and-resources/resource-library/state-patient-safety-and-quality-australian-hospitals-2019
[†]   HACs list complications only
[‡]   Public hospitals only, and all care types
[§]   Projected based on 2016–2017 National Hospital Cost Data Collection

Obviously, this type of data relies on many factors, but even if you halved the figures, on average, approximately four to six people out of every 100 hospital admissions have an adverse outcome.

These types of findings reinforce my advice to patients to take responsibility for the areas of their treatment that they can influence, and to check and recheck medication doses, possible side effects and contraindications with other medications.

This includes looking after your own cleanliness and hygiene to minimise the risk of infection and germs often found in hospitals. I constantly use the hand steriliser solution placed around the hospitals and avoid touching items in common areas where possible. If I do have contact with handrails, lift controls, etc., I wash my hands as soon as possible.

This advice is now essential and a part of daily life for not only cancer patients but for people in general since the outbreak of COVID-19.

Tip Number 11

Work with the nurses and doctors but if things are going badly, identify the problem and have it rectified as soon as possible.

Sometimes, the actions of the nursing staff are simply inexplicable.

I give below a few examples of some interesting decisions made during my many hospitalisations.

Hip surgery

After a hip replacement surgery, I had to arrange suitable transport from the hospital to home or I was advised that I would need an ambulance. My surgeon advised me not to bend my knee beyond 90 degrees as this might adversely affect the new artificial hip.

I arranged for my wife to collect me from the hospital in our 4WD, which was a suitable vehicle. While she was waiting downstairs, I was to be discharged and accompanied from the private hospital by a nurse.

When the nurse arrived, she told me it was hospital policy that all discharging patients leave in a wheelchair accompanied by a nurse.

Unfortunately, the only wheelchair available at the time was a child's wheelchair and she attempted to help me get into it.

I am six foot tall and getting into a child's wheelchair bent my leg upwards above 90 degrees, hurt my hip and left me in an uncomfortable and stupid position.

I promptly got her to help me out of the wheelchair and

advised her that she had just hurt my hip and told her that I would be walking out on crutches.

The nurse accompanied me down four levels of the hospital and into the discharge area, wheeling the useless child's wheelchair alongside me.

Night sweats

On another occasion in the same hospital, I was experiencing post-anaesthetic night sweats, rigours, chills and fevers (also known as post-anaesthetic shivering) at 3 am, and was lying in sheets that were soaked with perspiration.

It took almost an hour for the nurse on duty to come to my room after I pressed the call button. Her explanation was that she 'hated night duty' as they were understaffed, and she was having 'a bad night with a lot of sick patients'. When I discussed some of my issues with her and stated that these issues were on my file, she said, "We never get time to read patient files."

I told her that it was her bloody job to care for sick patients at night, that if she didn't like it then she should choose another vocation and if she was not coping, then she should seek assistance.

I also reminded her that I was being charged over $3,000 a night to stay in the hospital and expected better care in the future. She needed to read my file and understand why I was still in care and what my requirements were.

I was not there to make friends, but what I discovered is that often the squeaky wheel gets the oil and if you don't stick up for yourself then you will probably stay at the back of the queue.

On another occasion when I was in the surgical ward, I experienced a severe case of rigours and chills. A nurse was in the room and she assisted me and tried to keep me from falling out of the bed (yes, the rigours were that bad).

I held her so tightly that I left fingermarks on her arm while in the throes of the convulsions. I was shaking uncontrollably and asked her to put blankets on me to stop the chills. She argued and said that patients experiencing these symptoms were not to be warmed up as this could be dangerous.

I was in real distress and just said to her, "Give me a blanket now and don't argue with me!"

She supplied the blanket and I gradually warmed up until the chills and rigours stopped.

It took two nurses to hold me on the bed and prevent injury. Without their assistance I would have suffered even more.

The thing that disturbed me was the lack of knowledge and treatment for my condition.

Anyone who has had uncontrollable rigours and chills

two days after major abdominal surgery with a collapsed lung will understand my frustration, because the research I had done online from previous surgeries clearly states that first-line treatment for post-anaesthetic shivering is to warm the patient, and if no improvement occurs or the conditions worsen to administer pethidine, clonidine and nefopam.

I was given two Endone and two Panadol tablets, which helped at the time.

I apologised to the nurse for hurting her with my grip and for being so assertive, but also expressed concern why a nurse on the surgical ward did not know how to treat my very common symptoms. I showed her on my phone the online advice which clearly stated the opposite of her suggested treatment, which had made my condition worse at the time.

On the one hand, I can understand that her main focus was my care in relation to the major surgeries – stage 4 CCRC in my right kidney and a stage 2 CCRC in my left kidney – and associated complications, but on the other hand her general knowledge and nursing skills were in my view not at the required standard.

I owe my life to the surgeon/s who performed the surgeries and the medical and nursing staff who cared for me during and after my illnesses and procedures.

I have nothing but respect for the professions these individuals have chosen and the work they perform, but on occasion as I demonstrate through this book, lapses in practical knowledge and application are common and can quickly become serious and occasionally life threatening.

Ignoring an alarm

I was in one surgical ward where a person in the room across the corridor from me was obviously seriously ill and lapsing in and out of consciousness or sleep.

An unfortunate consequence of this was that the oxygen monitor on his finger continually fell off with his movements and he was unaware that it had happened.

The problem was that each time an alarm sounded the nurses ignored it because they knew it was not cause for concern in his case.

I had no such choice, as I was in the room next door. While I sympathised with his plight, I had to endure the incessant beeping of his monitor day and night.

On the third night of getting almost no sleep because of this incessant alarm, I called a nurse in and asked why they could not just tape the finger clamp to his finger, or turn it off, as it was useless under the circumstances.

Her reply was that they were aware of the problem and I could have my door closed if that would help.

This is another example of a lack of practical actions and duty of care.

Lodging complaints

I never had bad relationships with hospital nursing staff and I always thanked them for their efforts when I left. However, I have made a number of formal complaints resulting from my stays in certain hospitals which have been investigated and, in my view, concluded satisfactorily.

The reason for lodging these complaints was not selfish, but to bring to the attention of the hospital and their staff their accountability to patients and responsibility for their actions.

In most cases, the head nurse would visit me and apologise for the lack of treatment or service that had occurred, but I got tired of apologies and would state that I did not seek apologies, I just wanted professional care and for people to do their job properly.

'Just rip it off'

The most significant complaint was following hernia surgery on my abdomen, when I had a large adhesive dressing on my stomach covering the site of the surgery.

I had advised the medical and nursing staff prior to the surgery that I suffered an acute allergy to Fixomull® Stretch adhesive surgical tape, and that removal required care and an adhesive remover named Remove It (common in all hospitals).

On the morning after the surgery, a nurse came to remove the dressing and I told her about my condition. She said not to be a baby and that she would just rip it off quickly.

She tried to rip off the dressing before I could prevent her from doing so and ripped my skin off my stomach, which caused excruciating pain and left exposed skin in two places the size of a man's fist.

Panic then ensued with the nurse aware that she had royally stuffed up. I swore loudly at her and she left to get help.

This then became a real issue as I had a dressing half removed over day-old surgery with large patches of skin ripped from the site surrounding the surgery. I was in genuine pain and the rest of the dressing had to be removed.

This was compounded by my frustration that the reaction to surgical tape and dressings was in my file and had been discussed with the nursing staff and surgeon, but had been ignored by this nurse.

The damage was so severe that two nurses were immediately sent from the burns ward to salvage the situation and treat my issues.

They were distressed when they saw the damage but were able to remove the dressing and the skin and apply soothing ointment to quell the pain.

This incident left me with permanent scarring, and I was

in unnecessary pain for two or three months after the surgery as a result of this unprofessional action.

It was only the hospital's diligent and prompt investigation into this incident and the implementation of their findings that prevented me from suing them for damages incurred.

Patient care

Unfortunately, from my discussions with healthcare providers and my personal experiences, it appears that the delivery of patient care has changed over the last 10 years. Nursing staff are now university trained and more focused on administration and issues associated with the delivery of drugs and treatment protocols rather than on patient care and comfort.

This is a contentious issue and one often disputed by nursing representatives, but patently aware to doctors and patients.

I have found nurses to be caring and helpful, but less focused on a patient as a person. Obviously, this varies depending upon where you are and who you are dealing with, but the old days of nurses spending time with patients and seeking to be aware of their needs and comfort seems to have been replaced by a more clinical and rushed attitude towards tasks. Also, their perceived professional status on occasion may inhibit their delivery of a more personal service.

The pressures of cost and big business are in my view moving more towards the 'production line' approach to patient care.

I stress again that these are my personal observations from the last 10 to 15 years. However, they accurately reflect my experiences.

Tests and biopsies

When you are confronted by painful or invasive tests, biopsies, scans, etc., I suggest contacting the establishment beforehand and seeking details about the procedure and what it entails.

On one occasion during the kidney cancers, a kidney biopsy was required to map the kidney being operated on in the first surgery.

I was advised that this involved a procedure where I would be placed in an MRI machine and monitored by a medical team. They would insert a local anaesthetic in stages through my abdomen, closely followed by a biopsy needle until they reached my kidney where portions of the kidney would be taken.

I was also advised that most people chose to use a light general anaesthetic for this procedure, as it was very uncomfortable. In that situation, an overnight stay in the centre was possible.

I chose not to have the general anaesthetic and to rely on the local anaesthetic so that I could go home not long after the procedure.

There were two reasons for this decision:

1. I have had so many general anaesthetics that I wanted to avoid another one if possible
2. I have had so many medical procedures and tests that I was confident I would be able to meditate and endure the process. (I will cover meditation and stress relief in Chapter 7 of this book.)

The procedure was arduous and painful, and the medical and nursing staff at the facility were caring and exceptionally professional.

The doctor had arranged for a light general anaesthetic to be administered if I found the process too painful, so I had a backup plan.

The doctor was surprised at my ability to lower my blood pressure and remain calm through this procedure. When it was over (after about 45 minutes), he visited me in the recovery room specifically to congratulate me on the way I had managed the procedure. He said that no one in his experience had had the procedure and remained calm and perfectly still while pieces of their kidney were being removed.

I must add that I had my moments during the procedure,

especially when the needle hit the kidney and I was overcome by nausea and nearly blacked out.

I achieved my objectives though because I went home an hour after the procedure.

Once again, I controlled as much of the process as I could, knowing that the biopsy was essential for the mapping of the surgery. I was prepared to do whatever was necessary to complete the test.

All treatments carry some risk, and all treatments involve several parties and professionals, but as a patient it is essential that you remain the main player.

In my medical diary, I recorded the different tests and treatments I was undergoing and monitored my progress, which enabled me to have a more informed discussion with the treating GP and specialists.

I believe that it is important to understand the possible negative outcomes and processes that may form part of treatment, and then focus on the positive message. It's a tough race to get to the other end, and there are bound to be some tough times.

My view of any treatment at the time was that it was simply a means to an end, and I trusted the clinicians to do their job. My job was to:

- stay focused
- take the required medication

- continue to research my condition, treatment and medication and any developments that might be relevant to me
- stay as fit and healthy as possible
- avoid negative thinking and catastrophising possible future events by focusing on what positive outcomes were possible
- not give ground to poor treatment and/or incompetence which would jeopardise my health
- have a 'Plan A' and a 'Plan B' and if they both failed, quickly come up with a 'Plan C'.

In my view, the attitude of the patient is crucial to the outcome of any treatment. I tried out my dad jokes an all comers and tried to maintain my sense of humour.

On occasion, nursing staff wondered if I was completely mad, probably based on reasonable observations.

Once, while I was having the stem cell collection and sitting in the apheresis chair with long steel needles in each arm and the machine huffing and puffing while surrounded by morose nursing and laboratory staff, I was in fits of laughter and my movements caused the machine to shut down about four times, as no movement is allowed.

The reason I was laughing was because I had my phone loaded with podcasts and downloads of some of the most politically incorrect and controversial comedians that I could find. With my earphones in and my eyes closed, I imagined myself at their concerts and was having a great time.

The comedians' sometimes controversial content kept me amused for the four long and uncomfortable sessions in that chair. I stayed positive rather than reflecting on the facts: I felt terrible, looked shocking, had stage 4 cancer, was having my blood washed and separated, stem cells were being collected and possibly I'd need a stem cell transplant at some time in the future – if I lived that long.

To gain the best possible outcome from treatment, in this case chemotherapy, I suffered from many uncomfortable and disturbing side effects such as nausea, lack of sleep from the steroid drugs, pain, tenderness in the joints and many other issues.

This was during the make or break period when things were indeed bleak. The light at the end of the tunnel seemed a long way away and looked more like a train coming straight at me.

The chemotherapy sessions were brutal. I had no hair left, my skin was pale, I lost about 10 kilos and I felt very ill.

This was the time when concentrating on positive outcomes and focusing on small achievements was crucial.

I meditated each day, and during the nights when I could not sleep, I also used Neuro-Linguistic Programming (NLP). It's hard to prove the benefits, but I am convinced that this technique greatly assisted in my recovery.

My version of NLP was to:

- find a quiet relaxing position, either sitting in a comfortable chair, lying on a bed or even sitting in the chemotherapy chair
- close my eyes and imagine the chemotherapy and/or any medication that I was taking entering my system
- visualise the medication seeking out damaged white blood cells and destroying those cells
- visualise the dead white blood cells being disintegrated and then imagine my bone marrow making and releasing new fresh white blood cells into my immune system
- visualise myself recovering, with hair and a ruddy complexion, participating in sports or other activities that I enjoyed.

When I could not sleep, this activity kept me sane and I was able to imagine these events in the most finite of details to pass the time positively, rather than lying in bed worrying why I could not sleep.

I used this technique throughout my treatments to aid my recovery, keep me focused on positive outcomes and stop myself from going barking mad.

In my view, too much complexity has been introduced to some of these techniques, so I am going to provide my version of these skills.

I did not go to the Himalayas and sit in a cave with a Buddhist monk to learn these techniques, nor did I attend classes or online courses.

Instead, I applied my own research to well-known techniques and practices which suited me and my level of knowledge.

I then stuck to anything that worked and practised it until the benefits increased and I was able to apply them when needed.

NLP is often defined as learning the language of your own mind and is closely linked to self-hypnosis. There is no doubt that when used often and applied diligently, it can improve and make positive changes in your life.

There are numerous techniques and aids available online to assist people who struggle to relax the mind and achieve a reasonable state of meditation.

There are online apps and videos that provide guided meditation and relaxation exercises, but essentially meditation is the process of practising measured breathing techniques and muscle relaxation to achieve a state of calm.

Even though I have been practising meditation for over 30 years, on occasion while I was in hospital or going through long chemotherapy treatments, I would put my earphones in, lie back and listen to classical music and other music such as Tibetan chants, Gregorian chants and crystal bowl chakra music.

This state of calm has proven beneficial outcomes which may reduce anxiety, lower blood pressure and aid healing processes.

I could not change the circumstances, but I could change how I viewed them.

A prime example of this technique and its benefits is that between 2004 and 2018, my tennis partner Len Yates (also a professional tennis coach and accomplished player) and I have won a gold medal in the Pan Pacific Masters Games men's doubles age events. In 2018, we received a silver medal.

We had an unbroken period of 14 years over seven competitions as winners of this event, which is held in Australia every two years.

We believe that no other men's doubles combination has been able to achieve this result in this event, and we are relatively confident that it will not be replicated by another pair over a similar 14-year period.

During this time, I was obviously undergoing various treatments and surgeries, but was able to maintain my tennis skills and fitness to a level which enabled this continued success.

This achievement remains one of my best motivators, and the continued pursuit of winning the event gave me something to look forward to for many years.

For readers who wonder how this was achieved, I set out below some of the strategies we used.

The first occasion was in 2008 when I was undergoing the second session of chemotherapy. I was in day eight, which is when the drugs kick in and the effects are horrendous. I was struggling with nausea, headaches, joint pain and many other symptoms, and I felt as if I had the worst hangover in the world.

We had won two gold medals in the previous Pan Pacific Masters Games in the men's doubles, and I was desperate to try and win again.

I had paid for the entry and was almost resigned to the fact that I was too sick to play, but on the day, I rang my tennis partner and said I wanted to give it a crack. If I was unable to continue, then we would just forfeit and go home.

I got off the bed, had a hot shower and got dressed in my tennis gear.

This made me feel marginally better. Mentally, I was as strong as I could be.

At the tennis courts we discussed our tactics and came up with a plan to maximise our strengths and hide our weaknesses.

Obviously, I was not up to running around all day in 35-degree heat, but we could not let our opponents know that, so we devised the following plan:

- I have a powerful left-handed swing serve so I would serve first and my partner would cross at the net whenever possible to limit the balls coming deep in the court to me.

- To limit my running, I would attack more, and no matter what, after I had hit two balls in any rally I was going to tee off and go for a winner.
- My partner would be ready to cross at the net and cover off any cross-court returns aimed at me.
- My partner would retrieve the balls when I was serving and hand them to me, while making out we were discussing tactics to save me from bending down and extra walking.
- We would not tell anyone that I was undergoing chemotherapy for cancer, and I kept my hat on at all times (or just swapped it for a dry one) so no one would see my bald head.
- I appeared to be the most aggressive player with the big serve and forehand weapons, so a lot of the play was directed away from me to my partner.

This strategy worked like a charm, and we cruised through the first day and won the group and then the final play-off for our first gold medal of the tournament, the men's doubles age 50-plus event.

I was shattered when I got home and went straight to bed, but got up again the next morning and went through the same routine to play in the combined age men's doubles.

I have been playing tennis most of my life at a high level, so the shots and the reflexes were fine. It was the endurance that was the problem, so I kept up with chocolate bars, jelly babies and pain medication. This was combined with our strategy of two shots, then going for a winner, along with aggressive play on my behalf and swift and frequent intervention by my partner at the net.

If net shots for me looked difficult, I would leave them where possible and allow them to go over my head for my partner to cover on the baseline and then move to cover the other side of the court.

At the end of the second day, we had won our way to the final to play for a second gold medal and some of my friends and family joined the crowd to watch the final.

By that stage I was feeling really bad. I had visible shakes and was quite fatigued, so before the final match I ate a full bag of jelly babies, and had some dark chocolate and some pain medication.

Sheer willpower and tenacity drove me as I had no idea whether this would be my last tennis tournament. It made me more determined to win.

It could not have been achieved without my tennis partner's help and strategic support, and I owe him greatly for his support over the years.

We won the final and earnt another gold medal.

Because I had lost weight during the treatment, I looked

outwardly quite lean and fit. When we came off after the final match, a number of players and spectators came and wished me well and good luck with my treatment.

These comments came as quite a shock to us as we had not told anybody about it so that I would not be targeted during the matches and forced to run around unnecessarily. Still, it appeared to have become common knowledge.

When I reached my friends and family group, I asked how the spectators had known about my condition. My adult daughter said that during the final match someone in the crowd said that I looked too young to be playing in the 50-plus event.

My daughter's reply to these comments still makes me laugh. She said, "Not only is he nearer 60 and playing down an age group because of the age of his partner, but he's in the middle of chemotherapy for stage 4 cancer and should be home in bed!"

Hence my struggle became common knowledge, but it was too late as we had finished playing by then.

We have continued to win in this prestigious event and sometimes I have been well and sometimes not.

We combine well together as tennis players and laugh about our many victories.

We train hard and practise before these events and it has been one of the greatest achievements of my life to continue to play well and win at this prestigious event.

I have used the anticipation of defending our titles as positive reinforcement and something to look forward to every two years.

This is more about the power of the mind and what motivation and willpower can achieve than winning a tennis trophy.

The alternative would have been lying in bed sick and depressed because I was unable to play in the events when I was undergoing my various treatments.

I have no doubt that making the effort to get up and have a go helped me deal with the treatment and all of the nasty side effects.

But when I came home, I crashed for three days and stayed in bed until I recovered.

The reason for retelling these experiences in this book is not to wow you with my sporting prowess, but to realistically portray the measurable benefits of actions over choosing to stay in bed feeling terrible and facing negative thoughts and time which seems to drag. It's about doing something positive, doing something that makes you happy and that gets you out of bed.

It also proved to me the absolute power of the mind and body to overcome the most extreme pain and sickness.

In my case, the transition from lying in bed drooling on the pillow to getting up, having a hot shower, getting dressed and driving to the tennis courts took my mind off my predicament and stirred up positive feelings and adrenaline.

It was hard to focus on misery when I had two men at the other end of the tennis court firing tennis balls at me, and then the absolute elation of winning the gold medal despite my condition.

These victories over the years have built up my confidence and given me great internal strength that I have drawn on while undergoing procedures, treatments and medications.

No matter how bad I have felt at the time, the medals are still hanging on my study wall and I am planning my attack of the next event.

I realise not everybody can replicate my experiences, but my advice is to try not to lie in bed feeling sick and sorry for yourself.

There is a real risk of falling into this hole because the negative thoughts are in some cases true. You may well have a dire diagnosis, or be undergoing uncomfortable treatments, surgery or depression.

You may also be surrounded by people who lament your condition and provide you with sympathy and care, and it can be easy to lie in bed and say, "I have cancer, I may not live, I feel terrible, I have more treatments, surgeries or radiation to look forward to and life sucks."

Again, this may all be true, but the choice is either to surround yourself with these feelings, or to get up and get moving and do some sort of activity that takes your mind off negative thoughts and aids your recovery.

Tip Number 12

Do whatever you can to get moving and stay positive and motivated. Get a buddy and do things together. Chat online or talk about your issues, goals and achievements.

Record all of these things in your medical journal.

Chapter 5

Medication, Effects and Side Effects during and after Treatment

One of the most significant issues to deal with during cancer treatments are the side effects of chemotherapy and associated drugs.

I suggest that patients keep records of their past medical history and medications they are taking prior to commencing their treatment.

Most doctors check these details before commencing your treatment, but having a detailed list in your medical diary helps the process and may prevent contraindications with other medicines. Include any health supplements and powders and herbal supplements you are taking.

For example, grapefruit and grapefruit juice can interact with some medications listed below:

- Some cholesterol medications
- Some blood pressure medications
- Some heart rhythm medications
- Some anti-infection medications
- Several mood medications
- Some blood thinners
- Several pain medications
- Some erectile dysfunction and prostate medications
- Some antihistamines.

This is long list of increased side effects caused by such a common fruit. It shows the need for patients to conduct their own research into the medications they are taking, what may be prescribed and any possible contraindications and/or side effects, and discuss them with their treating clinicians.

During my treatments, I experienced the following side effects, some of which remain with me today:

Loss of taste and smell

This condition has remained with me and is unlikely to improve in my case. It is annoying, but as with most of these side effects it is better than being dead. I do remember what food used to taste like though, and quite often it helps to imagine what something used to taste like while eating, as it works to a degree.

The loss of smell does present some rather unique

problems. I have discovered that I need someone to check cooking appliances and BBQ gas bottles after I have used them as I cannot smell burning food or gas bottles left on.

This condition also occurs in the kitchen using other cooking apparatus and has caused a few anxious moments at home.

Once while we were camping in North Queensland, I cooked breakfast on the small BBQ hooked up to our caravan and then we went fishing.

On our return to the campsite a few hours later, the first thing my wife noticed was the strong smell of gas, so we quickly turned off the gas that I had left on and made sure no one lit a match for a while.

This could have been very dangerous to us and others.

I have discovered what foods have some taste for me and I savour them, but with other foods I have adopted the attitude that food is an essential part of life, and if I cannot taste it then I might as well consume healthy food as often as possible.

Unfortunately, the foods I can partially taste are high in fat and sugar, with chocolate being the main offender, so it is a constant battle to regulate my daily intake of this treat.

Another issue with the lack of taste is that I find drinking water as my only form of beverage is boring beyond belief and sometimes, I crave the taste of other drinks.

I said previously that after almost 17 years of no alcohol

and no red meat, after chemotherapy treatments I had cravings for red meat, but the alcohol was a different story.

I was not willing to break such a long abstinence, however one day after my treatment had ceased, someone at my golf club bought a round of beers after a game. I took a sip of mine and discovered that I could taste the bitterness of the beer.

This was a real revelation. Although good for me, my wife lost her designated driver and I had 17 years of credit to call in.

As beer and straight spirits such as tequila and scotch deliver the most taste to me, obviously I have to carefully manage it. If I consumed these drinks every day, things would go downhill rapidly.

I treat these outcomes as a sign from above that some pleasures remain after the treatment.

After four or five days of meals that I am unable to taste, I often reach for a beer at the end of the day. As this can be a bad habit to get into, I now purchase low and/or zero alcohol beer which provides the tastes that I require without the consumption of alcohol.

Meals like chicken, veal, turkey, fish and other relatively bland foods have no taste for me at all, but strong sauces and chillies when added to these food groups can liven them up.

With reduced taste sensations, it can also be a trap to add too much salt to meals, chasing that extra bit of taste. If you suffer a loss of taste after treatments, my advice is to try as many different foods as possible and find what you can taste (if anything). If not, eat healthily and not just for the sake of eating.

Peripheral neuropathy

This is the loss of feeling in the extremities, such as fingers and toes, as well as tingling and burning in these locations at night. This condition has not improved greatly since the treatment and is an unfortunate side effect of some of the chemotherapy drugs. I still play golf and tennis and walk without much hindrance. I make sure that I wear shoes with cushioned inserts and almost never go barefoot.

Exercise and the daily use of a shakti mat (spiky massage mat) have increased the feeling in my feet. The feeling in my fingertips is very slowly improving.

I once had acupuncture, having told the practitioner of my peripheral neuropathy in the soles of my feet and the tingling and nerve damage from the chemotherapy. His answer was to insert a needle in the sole of my foot to see how far the damage went and where the undamaged nerves were. My advice here is to never let anyone do that to you.

Despite the nerve damage, it was excruciatingly painful and in the end, after three or four treatments with the acupuncturist trying his best, there was no improvement.

Loss of hair (which does usually grow back)

Most people's hair grows back after the completion of chemo-therapy treatments. However, it can come back a different colour and a different consistency. Eyebrows, pubic hair and whiskers also usually return after a while.

Cravings for nicotine, alcohol and food

After 28 years of not smoking, the cancer drugs and steroids stimulated this unnatural craving. Most doctors do not warn you about it in detail, probably because it does not affect all patients and if it does it affects people differently.

One of the most commonly prescribed steroid drugs is prednisone. I was prescribed large doses of this drug to reduce inflammation and suppress (lower) the body's immune response. I was advised that the drug might make me a bit restless and hyperactive.

Other medication often included in chemotherapy infusions are dexamethasone and anti-anxiety drugs. Prednisone and dexamethasone are synthetic (man-made) corticosteroids (steroids) used for suppressing the immune system and inflammation.

These drugs have effects similar to other corticosteroids such as triamcinolone (Kenacort), methylprednisolone (Medrol), and prednisolone (Prelone).

To say these drugs may cause some anxiety and agitation

is, in my view, like saying that cutting off your legs may impede your ability to run a marathon.

The cravings associated with prednisone were in my case extreme, to the extent that my appetite for food was insatiable.

I did not recognise this as associated with the drug until by chance I was watching a television documentary where a young woman had put on 160 kilos and sought medical help to lose the weight.

The doctors discovered that she was being treated for non-Hodgkin lymphoma (same as me) and that the high doses of prednisone she was on were causing food cravings (same as me).

Until that time, I had no idea that the drug was the cause of my extreme hunger pangs.

At one stage I was sitting in my leather lounge chair considering having a chew of it to see if there was any meat left on the leather.

Most people reading this comment would not believe that someone of sound mind could even contemplate such an action.

I am living proof that my appetite was out of control. I would often eat a full chicken for lunch followed by a cake and some chocolates, and be ready to eat again in two hours.

I rarely felt satiated, no matter how much food I consumed.

I knew from my previous training regime that this craving was not normal. Combined with my research on prednisone after watching the documentary about the young woman who gained all the weight, I took steps to stop the consumption of food.

My way of dealing with it was to treat the hunger pangs as a confrontation and fight against the cravings.

I restricted my food intake drastically, to the extent that I made a can of beef and vegetable soup my go-to evening meal.

I stopped reactive eating and consuming large meals and snacks.

The cravings remained while I was on the drugs, but I successfully managed them and when the drugs stopped the cravings stopped.

The other demon drug that affected me badly was dexamethasone.

Each person reacts in their own way to certain drugs, but dexamethasone caused me many problems during my treatments. My experience is one of the main reasons why I stress in this book to do your research and be prepared for possible side effects of drugs and treatments.

My cravings for food, alcohol and cigarettes went off scale when I was on prednisone and dexamethasone.

Shortly after my first chemotherapy infusion and associated drugs, I craved red meat and alcohol for the first time in 17 years. I took to both with a vengeance, and continue to do so.

One of the things to be considered in relation to these drugs is that people can only base their feelings and behaviours on past experiences and illnesses.

When you have poison and steroid drugs chemically administered, your system is unsure what is going on and reactions can vary greatly between people.

Many of the effects of these drugs are not 'normal'. They introduce feelings and symptoms never experienced before.

In my case, cravings were exaggerated, and I needed to recognise them as being drug related and manage them to minimise damage.

It does appear that I have a low tolerance to caffeine and other stimulants and for this reason I generally avoid coffee and caffeinated drinks.

On large doses of prednisone and dexamethasone, I found it almost impossible to sleep, and my temper and anger levels were off scale.

These changes were so severe that I took steps to remove my firearms from the house. I told my family that I was struggling to control such violent temper reactions to the most minor events. I explained that it was the drugs, not me, but it was real, and I was concerned that my anger would result in violence.

I told them to walk away if I started shouting or reacting

angrily to comments or actions, and not to confront me if possible.

At the time, I was playing golf at my golf club regularly with two doctors, one of whom remains my treating GP. The other doctor was facing his own cancer battle and was also taking prednisone and other drugs.

Our temper tantrums were often on display, and we advised other members, "We are on medication. Don't be offended."

On one Saturday morning competition, I hit a poor drive off the 11th tee and got so angry that I threw my 1-wood further than I hit the ball. The throw was so good that my $700 1-wood sailed over the boundary fence next to the fairway.

To this day, I wonder how I had the strength to throw it that far. I had to go and retrieve the club, with the members behind us waiting to tee off watching in amusement. The most embarrassing thing was that one of the members who had witnessed a very unprofessional display of anger from me was a client of mine.

I also had hallucinations on occasion, with visions of psychedelic images and shapes. I discussed these occurrences with my haematologist, who asked me how I dealt with them. I replied that I knew it was the drugs and not real, and that they would go away eventually.

He said that it was not unusual to have hallucinogenic

reactions like these while on doses of the medication that I was taking.

Armed with this information, I considered it part of the treatment and tried to get through each day and night as best I could.

My battle with dexamethasone, though, became serious and life threatening during my stem cell collection process. I detail this struggle below to demonstrate the minefield that cancer patients may face during their treatment and how I dealt with it.

This is a warts and all summary, and one of the reasons I was prompted to write the book.

* * * * *

Stem cell collection

Approximately 12 months after my chemotherapy treatments ceased, I was given the option of a stem cell collection for storing my stem cells in case the cancer returned and I needed further treatment.

A bone marrow transplant using my own stem cells (autologous transplant) is more effective, obviously, because they are my own stem cells, not from a donor, and so they do not require any anti-rejection drugs.

These transplants use healthy bone marrow which

produces blood cells, including the white blood cells that are crucial to your immune system.

Blood cancers damage bone marrow, and so do chemotherapy and radiation treatments.

A stem cell transplant allows new stem cells to take over from your damaged bone marrow so that your body can produce healthy, cancer-free blood cells.

The process for this involves an initial chemical infusion treatment, to move blood-forming stem cells from your bone marrow to your bloodstream. Stem cell collection is performed in hospital.

A preliminary conditioning treatment is required where the patient is administered doses of chemotherapy or radiation to kill the existing stem cells and the cancer cells. Once this occurs, your immunity is destroyed, and the new stem cells can begin to grow.

I am not going to explain all the medical issues associated with this procedure, but the stem cell collection process was brutal and nearly killed me.

I document my experiences in this book so that readers can see the type of situations that arise, and how they need to be evaluated and dealt with.

The first issue arose with the full-day infusion in hospital to commence the process. The infusion of chemicals was combined with multiple saline solution infusions and my body started to swell almost straightaway.

The goal of this process was to make my body neutropenic, which means to reduce the white blood cell count. White blood cells fight infection through the immune system, so becoming neutropenic destroys the immune system and leaves the patient susceptible to infection, which can be life threatening.

I also had two injection ports inserted into my lower abdomen for four-hourly injections of a drug to promote growth of bone marrow. This drug and the associated process caused extreme swelling, pain and discomfort in my long bones and needed to be managed through prescribed pain medication.

My specialist advised me to religiously take the pain medication so as not to allow the pain to take hold. If it did, there was little they could then do to ease the pain.

This becomes important as the tale continues.

The chemicals made me very unwell and nauseated and my stomach swelled alarmingly.

After the infusion, I spent a night in hospital and left to go home for a few days. From there, I would go from the Gold Coast to a private hospital in Brisbane for the stem cell collection.

My oncologist gave me a prescription for the medications I needed for this period, and we filled it at the hospital pharmacy. It was a large package of medicines, including injections and a list of instructions.

Unfortunately, I encountered a trainee nurse who did not speak English well. She told me that she did not think I needed the prescription pain medication as it was very high strength, so she had not included it in my medication.

When we got home, I checked the instructions which specifically stated that the pain medication was crucial to the treatment and must be used as directed.

I rang the hospital and checked with a senior nurse who agreed that the prescribed pain medication was required. She apologised for the mistake.

My wife then had to leave me and drive to the hospital to pick up the medication.

I wrote a formal complaint to the hospital about the nurse who had made a decision beyond her capabilities that could have had dire consequences for me, compounded by her limited ability to communicate to me in English and to perform her job competently as she made other mistakes while treating me. This was not a vindictive act. I wanted the hospital to be aware that this young inexperienced nurse had placed me in a very serious predicament.

The hospital replied to my complaint with the results of their investigation and advised that the nurse had been reprimanded for her actions and sent for retraining.

While I was at home following this infusion, I did not sleep and was seriously unwell. When I went to the hospital in Brisbane, I was agitated, had not slept for three days and was hallucinating.

I knew on the first day in the private hospital that it was going to be tough when they wheeled another bed into my private room, pulled the dividing curtain across and admitted a new patient.

This patient was also neutropenic and awaiting a similar stem cell collection to me, but he was very ill with a cold or virus and was coughing and sneezing.

I heard the doctor tell him to spit out mucus and blow his nose into the bathroom sink in the room to help his breathing.

At that stage, my immune system was compromised and any infection could have resulted in severe complications up to and including death. I had been told to stay away from people and had restricted visitors while in hospital.

My wife was with me at the time and we were horrified that they had placed me in this position and compromised my health so seriously.

I rang the nurses' bell and when they appeared, I blew up, reminding them of my condition. I told them that I was supposed to be in a private room and kept away from infection. It appeared that this had been forgotten by the nursing staff who had admitted the new patient.

They apologised, and said they were busy and had a lot of sick patients. My response was to tell them to get the sick person out of my room, or I would smother him while he was asleep and sue them after the process for negligence.

I was agitated and upset and hadn't slept for days and was not prepared to risk everything just because they were busy, and I let them know this in a very clear and precise manner.

They very quickly removed the patient from my room, cleaned up the area and apologised for the mistake.

The reason I am retelling this series of events is to demonstrate the need for the patient to be in control of circumstances when others are not performing their duties professionally and/or in your best interests.

I was really sick, depressed, anxious and worried about my future and the cancer, not to mention the thought of a stem cell transplant at some time in the future. The recent death of a friend of mine from a stem cell transplant was also playing on my mind.

I got through that day but was still unable to sleep and spent most of the night in the exercise room with another patient from the cardiac ward who was also an exercise junkie and could not sleep.

We worked the weights, exercise bike and rowing machine like demons, and then went to bed when the sun came up and the nurses started to roam around.

By then, I was thinking that the rodeo was not going well, and I was in serious trouble, surrounded by clowns not cowboys.

I was supposed to have four-hourly injections as part of the treatment to promote bone marrow growth, but they constantly forgot to come and administer them. Again, I rang the nurses' bell and asked why I was being forgotten.

Their response was understandable but not acceptable.

They told me that I was probably the fittest person in the cancer ward at the moment, and that they had a ward full of people who were literally dying, and they were stretched to the limit. They advised me that if I wanted clean linen, to get it from the storeroom myself. With the injections, they could not guarantee they would be administered every four hours as required.

They also advised that if I needed a shower or to use the bathroom, to do it without calling on the nurses to assist as I was able-bodied enough to carry out these functions unaided.

This left me in a pretty bad place, so I told them to bring the injections into my room and place them in the small fridge in the room and I would administer them myself. I did administer the injections myself into the injection ports in my abdomen, unaided by the nurses, and they hurt like hell.

That night I had serious hallucinations of little green men coming into my room trying to take me by the hand.

I had not had proper sleep for days, and I was so anxious, angry and hyper that I felt as though my heart was about to explode. I knew that I was in real trouble and at risk of serious injury if something was not done immediately about my problems.

I got up at 4 am and dressed in my street clothes. Then I approached the nurses' station and told the duty nurse that I had not slept for days, was having psychotic episodes and hallucinations, my treatment was not going as planned and I was at serious risk of collapsing from exhaustion and fatigue.

I demanded to see the head nurse and medical supervisor as soon as they were available, and suggested she look me up on the internet to check my extensive professional qualifications and background in workplace investigations, workplace health and safety and associated legal matters.

Apart from representing some of the largest corporations in the world at the time in industrial relations and conflict management (Exxon and Mayne Nickless), I also have post-graduate legal qualifications in arbitration and over 35 years of dealing with complex technical and legal matters.

I suggested she check me out online to assure her that I was not delusional and was someone to be reckoned with. In a calm and non-aggressive manner, I said that with my background and experience, unless I was able to meet with the head nurse and medical supervisor ASAP, I would be leaving the hospital immediately and going to the emergency ward of the nearest public hospital to seek treatment.

I asked her name and the name of the other nurses on

duty in the ward, explaining that I would be commencing legal action against them for negligence. My quote to her was that they would 'all be living in a cardboard box' by the time I finished the legal action against them.

This may seem extreme to the reader, but I was at the end of my endurance and sure that I was heading for a very bad outcome.

My fears were increased when I was informed that the patient I had been exercising with the night before had had a heart attack and died a few hours later.

At no time during the night did any nurses come into the gym and check on us. We had been left to our own devices.

I stayed in my street clothes and at about 8 am, the head nurse and doctor arrived together. The doctor asked me to sit down and relax, and I advised him that I was staying in my street clothes, was not going to sit down, would look him in the eyes and not allow a power imbalance to occur.

The doctor and nurse patiently listened to my concerns which I relayed to them in clear and concise terms. They said they had looked me up on the internet and understood that I was a highly qualified professional capable of carrying out the threat of legal action against them.

The meeting was cordial and professional. I reiterated that on top of all the other issues, I was seeing aliens, bright colours and shapes and losing my vision. In my view, I was suffering from psychotic episodes.

I also explained that I felt the drugs were making me violent and I was concerned for my safety and the safety of others. I told them I was trained in two forms of martial arts and they would need a SWAT mission to hold me down if nothing changed.

The doctor again asked me to sit down and stay as relaxed as possible, and he would return within an hour to discuss what to do.

I was reassured by his concern and commitment to find out what was going wrong.

About 30 minutes later, he returned with a nurse and asked me to listen to him as he was clear that he knew what the problem was. He had checked through my treatment and determined that at the hospital where I had the initial infusion, they had administered a dosage of dexamethasone three times what this hospital would normally administer for that treatment.

He advised that although this dosage was higher than the recommended dosage, it was still within allowable guidelines.

I had had an adverse reaction to the high dosage and was suffering from the effects.

He also stated my reaction to a dose of this size was not unusual, and quite often patients administered dosages less than I had received exhibited violent and bizarre behaviour and had trouble sleeping.

They were concerned about my reaction to the drug,

my lack of sleep and other symptoms, combined with my concerns about my treatment and care to date. They said my condition was serious, and I could face heart failure and/or other complications unless treated. They arranged for me to be immediately placed in an isolation critical care ward, where I would be treated and closely monitored.

I sincerely thanked them for hearing and understanding my condition and distress and agreed to their plan.

Four hours after this move, I started having full body spasms with excruciating pain in all the muscles of my body and particularly in my chest.

The nurses became increasingly concerned that my condition was deteriorating badly and called the consulting specialist for advice. It was 7 pm at the time.

His advice was that my condition was critical, and unless the seizures stopped, I would need to be placed in the cardiac critical care ward as a heart attack was imminent.

I will just return to the original intent here, which was for me to go to hospital for a stem cell collection. I was then in the throes of a steroid drug overdose, and in a critical condition facing heart failure after being neglected by the treatment providers.

I was in terrible pain, with the seizures coming every couple of minutes, each one leaving me more physically and mentally drained.

A nurse then came into my room and said the advice

from the consulting doctor was that the only way to stop my body's extreme reaction to the drug and the other associated issues was to knock me out for 12 hours with a strong sedative. This would allow my body to rest, calm the seizures and prevent heart failure.

I asked what other options there were and his response was, "None."

You can understand how low I felt at that moment. Based on past experiences, and facing the thought of being unconscious for 12 hours and relying on good care while I was under the medication, did not fill me with confidence.

I am also smart enough to realise when my options are limited to take the best one available, which was the only one, so I stuck out my arm and said, "Knock me out."

The loneliness and apprehension of not knowing whether I would wake up from that ordeal while I was lying in a hospital bed hours away from my family and friends can only be understood by people who have faced similar circumstances, but I am sure that you get the idea.

They certainly weren't joking, as I was unconscious almost immediately and woke up 12 hours later.

I was awake for less than 10 minutes the morning after these events, when a nurse came into the room and said that my stem cell collection appointment in the apheresis room was due in 30 minutes. She said if I was not able to be there in time, I would miss the appointment and they would assign the day session to another patient on the waiting list. Was this OK with me? Her advice was that before I got out of bed, I should wait until mid-morning to see the specialist after my ordeal of the night before.

I told her in no uncertain terms to ring them straight back and tell them I would be there in time, that it was not OK with me. The stem cell collection process was the reason I had been through so much suffering and I was not prepared to miss a session.

I was scheduled for four sessions and after each collection the stem cells would be sent to the laboratory for analysis and measurement.

Before the treatment, I had been told that the number of stem cells reduces after each session, and it is important to collect them before there are too few for collection.

I knew the seriousness of the collection process and timing, but the nurse had been quite happy for me to miss the second collection and upset the schedule and my bookings for future sessions by putting another patient into the procedure and leaving me in limbo.

I knew as soon as I woke up that the effects of the steroid drug had reduced. I had slept properly for the first time in two weeks and actually felt quite good.

If I had not felt so well, or I had believed I needed further help, I would have stayed in bed and missed the appointment.

I got up, had a shower, got dressed and rushed to the

apheresis room and commenced the treatment. I had to sit in a chair with long steel needles inserted into each arm and stay completely still for four or five hours while my blood was filtered and the stem cells collected.

When the procedure was completed, I was supposed to return to the ward I was assigned to, but it was mid-afternoon and I had had a pretty bad couple of days, so I zipped up my hoodie to hide the injection ports and tubes in my arms and left the hospital. I walked down to Southbank, an entertainment precinct in the city of Brisbane only a short distance from the hospital, had a nice afternoon tea and watched a free concert.

I then returned to the hospital. No one had even noticed that I was missing for three hours.

That whole ordeal nearly killed me, and if I did not have such a high-profile professional reputation and had not been willing to take control of my situation, I am sure that my complaints and my deteriorating conditions would have been ignored or discovered too late, with catastrophic outcomes.

Tip Number 13

If something is wrong, if your treatment or care is not being administered or it is neglected, deal with it, look after your care, don't become a statistic, make some noise!

Quite often, you are not advised when additional drugs and sedatives are added to the chemical infusion, and it is only when you ask the questions about additional drugs or you are aware of side effects that this information is provided.

* * * * *

Nausea

I found the anti-nausea drugs provided adequately dealt with nausea. You just need to be careful what you eat and when. I found that if I ate a food or had a drink that I particularly enjoyed straight after a chemotherapy treatment, I could no longer tolerate it the next time I had it. Once, my daughter brought me some luxury donuts after the infusion, which I consumed and then was violently ill. My body and mind associated the food with the reaction to the drugs, and all these years later, I cannot even look at a donut without feeling nauseated. I avoid eating any of my favourite foods while undergoing chemotherapy treatments.

Cravings and loss of appetite

If you have a craving for food, recognise it as a symptom of the drugs and deal with it as an issue.

Don't succumb to overeating. Manage your food intake.

This symptom was very difficult to deal with and was never mentioned to me by any medical staff. If you do some research, you will find that it is a common symptom associated with steroidal drugs.

Try and plan how you are going to manage the required intake of nutrition while maintaining a relatively healthy diet and exercise regime.

One of the issues can also be the loss of appetite associated with chemotherapy and even after surgery.

After my first partial nephrectomy surgery, I lost nine kilos in 10 days. This was simply because I did not feel like eating. All I could manage was a cup of soup and some small snacks a day.

I had to force myself to eat just to get nutrition back into my body, even though I did not feel hungry.

I was further freaked out when I had my first bowel movement after the surgery. This was assisted by high doses of laxatives to counteract the chronic constipation caused from the pain management drugs.

My stools were bright orange. I immediately looked online for an answer to this strange symptom and discovered that it was due to the massive doses of antibiotics I was taking to heal the collapsed lung and pneumonia that I was experiencing.

These conditions had occurred during my surgery from lying on my side for the four to five-hour procedure.

Again, I had to work this out for myself, but it was confronting at the time.

I stuck to my tried and tested practice of eating when I was hungry and eating anything that I craved and had some taste.

Lack of sleep

This is something that all patients going through treatment will have to deal with at some time, whether through discomfort from surgery, chemotherapy or radiation therapy, reaction to drugs or just plain anxiety.

I dealt with it by focusing on trying to stay calm, realising it was the drugs preventing my sleep and doing activities or watching TV until I felt tired enough to return to bed.

Short-term sleep medication may be an option during this phase of treatment, but it depends entirely on the individual and their medical circumstances.

I chose not to seek more medication and looked at it from the point of view that the treatment was needed to save my life and the effects would wear off eventually.

I just had to get through each second, minute and hour of the day and night as best I could and concentrate on the big picture.

Deep breathing, meditation and concentrating on positive thoughts were my best weapons at night. However, the impact of drug-induced insomnia and anxiety at night can be profound and should be managed to reduce negative impacts using whatever strategy helps at the time.

Tip Number 14

Lack of sleep can be upsetting for spouses and family members also living in the house. They should be made aware of your discomfort, how you are dealing with it and how they may be able to help.

Hallucinations/delirium

Hopefully, you will not experience this symptom, but if you do, remember that it is usually the drugs. Raise it as soon as possible with your doctor, and discuss how to deal with this disturbing side effect of certain drugs and steroids.

I experienced flashes of colour, strong dark lines and shapes (like Tetris) when I closed my eyes, and as mentioned previously on occasion saw figures and images that clearly were not real.

The difficult part is knowing how to recognise what is real and not real when you are taking a cocktail of strong drugs and chemicals.

Lack of sleep, drugs, anxiety, fatigue, medical procedures, the pressures of daily life all create an environment where your mental state can be fragile. It is important to recognise that many of these symptoms are part and parcel of what you are going through and will improve over time. It is essential that you stay focused on completing the treatment and coming out the other side.

Flashes of anger and anxiety

From my experiences and my discussions with other cancer patients, increased irritation and anger often occur during treatment due to the chemicals and drugs used, particularly steroids like prednisone and dexamethasone.

Each person has their own coping measures for dealing with emotions and reactions. My advice is to look out for any deviations in your normal behaviour, and try and stay as rational and as calm as possible. See this increased anxiety as part of the treatment and drugs and as something that will go away in time.

Do not underestimate the intensity of the flashes of anger that these drugs can cause and be prepared to recognise the symptoms and deal with them.

'Roid rage' is real and scary, and even today I clearly remember the ease with which I had anger outbursts and how difficult they were to control at the time.

Warn your friends and family that outbursts of anger may occur. I found apologising in advance lightened up the situation somewhat.

Weight loss

A lot of people also lose their appetite while on certain chemo-therapy drugs or immediately after surgery or radiation treatment, which has the effect of dramatic weight loss.

I dealt with this symptom during the treatment by eating whenever I felt hungry and whatever I felt like at the time.

If I craved a food, I ate it, because most of the time during the chemotherapy or after surgery I was nauseated and turned off by the idea of food.

My way of dealing with it was to take nutrition when I could.

After surgery, it was similar although different. Your body and bodily functions slow down for a long period under the anaesthetic, and it takes some time for the organs to start working again (the bowels especially).

My go-to breakfast and how I got nutrition quickly with-out sitting down and eating meals was a smoothie made up of the following ingredients:

- 1 handful frozen berries
- 1 handful mixed unsalted nuts
- 1 tablespoon plain yoghurt
- 1 banana (can be changed to another main ingredient if daily)
- 1 cup steel cut rolled oats
- 2 tablespoons organic protein powder (if allowed: after my kidney cancer this item was removed)
- 4 pitted fresh dates

If it was later in the day or evening and I did not feel like eating, I would have a green smoothie with the following ingredients:

- Broccoli
- 1 or 2 Brussels sprouts
- Celery
- A whole tomato
- A splash of Tabasco sauce (optional)
- 2 radishes
- Raw spinach leaves

These recipes worked for me, because sometimes I could not face a full cooked meal. Still, I knew I needed to keep up a nutritional food source to allow my body to heal and address my rapid weight loss and constipation after both chemotherapy and surgery.

I also added a tablespoon each of fibre and inulin to these drinks.

Swollen stomach

After the first two chemotherapy infusions, my stomach swelled alarmingly. This also affected my eating habits, as I felt uncomfortable after consuming only a small amount of food.

Swelling or edema is quite common during chemotherapy treatments and is generally associated with fluid retention. It may also be the more serious condition known as paralytic ileus, a condition where there is a blockage that prevents the passage of intestinal contents even though there is no actual obstruction.

This latter condition can be very serious and if left untreated can cause tissue death and intestinal tear or a life-threatening infection of the abdominal cavity.

Sometimes when cancer spreads to the abdominal lining, it can cause irritation, stimulating the lining and creating extra fluid, which results in the swelling of the stomach.

A large amount of saline solution is flushed through your body while undergoing treatment and in my view, this aids the fluid retention and swelling.

There have been cases of patient's internal organs exploding while undertaking chemotherapy treatment, so it is not to be underestimated.

There are so many reasons why stomach swelling may occur during cancer treatment, so it is important to advise your doctor as soon as the symptoms appear.

Tips for dealing with stomach swelling include:

- Walking
- Avoiding standing for long periods
- Eating a balanced diet
- Yoga
- Massage
- Avoiding tight clothing
- Reducing salt intake
- Taking peppermint capsules (check with your doctor).

Anaemia

I looked for advice from my doctor on this issue. I also researched that beetroot was useful for strengthening the body's power to regenerate and reactivate the red blood cells which supply the body with fresh oxygen and help reduce anaemia. I also have lean red meat at least once a week and eat a lot of broccoli and beans.

I incorporated beetroot and beetroot juice into my diet as a result of this research, and up to date my red blood cell count is within normal range and has been for over five years.

Constipation

This common but uncomfortable side effect of cancer treatment I found was successfully treated by laxative products that are commercially available from the chemist.

One tip I got from a helpful nurse was to take more than the dose recommended for normal use while undergoing chemotherapy treatment, as the digestive system was under different stressors.

I cannot advise anybody to take more than the prescribed or recommended dosage of any substance, but I will say, it worked for me.

This is a real issue and often overlooked in hospital initially, so during latter treatments I requested a laxative early based on my previous experiences.

Many of the opioid drugs used to treat and manage pain, combined with long periods under anaesthetic during surgery, create a perfect storm for constipation. With so many other issues relating to your condition, your bowel movements can be forgotten.

It is not everybody's favourite topic, but if left too long it can be serious and impede your recovery.

Lying prone for long periods of time does not help this condition and if possible, drinking lots of fluid and trying to spend some time standing up and/or walking can help.

Fatigue

Fatigue management will be an issue for anyone undergoing radiation, chemotherapy or surgery or a combination of all three.

It is a difficult aspect of the treatment because everyone has a different level of fitness and general health prior to commencing the treatment. Diet, fitness history, genetics and willpower can all have an effect on fatigue and fatigue management.

While I stress the importance of staying positive and focused on positive outcomes, often things are quite dire, with medical issues, treatment issues, family issues and a general malaise that comes with dealing with the plethora of matters that a person facing this type of ordeal has to deal with.

It is not as simple as taking a pill, or 'pulling your socks up'. Quite often, you have dark days and they are hard to deal with.

Cancer patients are often not able to participate in vigorous exercise. Lack of sleep or too much sleep and lying around for days on end can make you feel more tired and less willing to exercise when you are able.

Surgery is a whole different set of circumstances and requires a range of methodologies to help recuperate after the event.

Over the last 10 years, I have had the following surgical procedures:

- Abdominal hernia correction
- Left hip full replacement
- Right hip full replacement
- Umbilical hernia correction
- Right kidney partial nephrectomy
- Left kidney partial nephrectomy.

The recovery from each of these surgeries was different, but the process was fairly similar.

Exercise is generally minimal for the first four to six weeks and then after that, providing there are no complications, a gradual return to physical exercise is possible. For sports such as golf, this is generally after six to eight weeks and for tennis, approximately six months.

A return to more physical contact sports depends upon the individual and their specific medical advice.

Mouth and throat ulcers

Following my first chemotherapy session, I developed severe mouth and throat ulcers that made swallowing difficult and were painful 24 hours a day. This was another reason I had smoothies and soup during the chemotherapy treatment periods.

I did not pay too much attention to these ulcers as they would come and go, and I had other bigger issues to worry about.

It wasn't until two years later when undergoing the stem cell collection that a nurse told me to use a mouthwash as a gargle before and after each meal. This consists of around one litre of warm water with one teaspoon of bicarbonate of soda and one teaspoon of salt.

This small tip reduced the symptoms dramatically, and I am indebted to her for that advice.

I blame myself for not researching this side effect at the time, as once I did some research it was clearly identified as a side effect of the chemotherapy drugs in some patients.

It is also quite common in cancer patients who are undergoing radiation treatment to the head, neck or chest.

It would have been nice for someone to have advised me earlier to expect this issue and provide some preventative advice such as the mouthwash.

Other side effects of chemotherapy and other cancer treatments

- Weakened immune system.
- Bleeding.
- Hearing issues.
- Loss of libido.

- Effects on fertility in women.
- Skin and nail issues.
- Swollen hands and feet.

After my first hip replacement surgery, I was placed on the following pain management drugs immediately following the surgery and while still in hospital:

- Morphine: administered through a patient-controlled analgesia (PCA) mechanism set up in the hospital ward by the pain management specialists. This system allowed me to administer pain relief on an as-needed basis. This was in conjunction with the other pain medication being administered orally
- Endone: two to four every four hours
- Panadol: two every four hours.

For the second hip replacement surgery, I was placed on similar drugs and dosages but had some disturbing side effects that continued throughout my surgeries and recovery periods.

However, the morphine was replaced by fentanyl which in my view was less effective and less pleasant.

In my experience there is an increased reluctance in some hospitals to use morphine and morphine derivatives, due to their addictive traits, for post-operative pain management.

My view as a patient who has had high doses of all of these

drugs, as opposed to the clinicians who make the decisions, is simply that morphine, heroin, oxycodone and pethidine provide the best pain relief with accompanying feelings of euphoria. There is no doubt in my view that they are better for pain management, general well-being and recovery.

Obviously, this is based only on my experiences and my medical conditions and it is a general observation only.

The first time I had a hit of morphine from the PCA after surgery, the lack of any pain at all and the instant hit of euphoria was a feeling that made me understand after all my time on this planet why drug addiction is so prolific, and why people would chase this feeling.

My views however are blunter than this. If you are recovering in hospital after surgery or you are in acute pain, then these drugs should be in play. Hospitals are not back alley drug dens, and should not be treated as such. Once the initial use of the drugs is complete, they should be decreased and eventually stopped and the patient not sent home with repeat prescriptions which may lead to addiction.

I struggle with the concept that patients may not get the best pain medication available. In my view, this is because the rest of the world and governments in general cannot deal with the levels of substance abuse and opioid addiction present in the community.

While I accept that addiction in its many forms is recognised as a disease, there are also choices to be made in some circumstances, and to continue to take strong pain-killing medicine when it is required – following surgery, chemotherapy or other serious medical conditions – is necessary, but to continue to take them is in my view a choice made by the individual.

Progressing to stronger drugs like methamphetamines and heroin is a choice at the first level, and then the addiction kicks in and the serotonin receptors in the brain are changed, feeding the addiction and becoming a disease.

It is also my view, as controversial as it may be, that people need to take responsibility for their own actions and apply real strength, willpower and common sense to their decisions in relation to the use and abuse of prescription medication.

What a lot of people do not understand is that the drugs most commonly associated with addiction provide numbness, euphoria and are essentially one of the most pleasurable feelings available. When users chase this feeling and the dosages increase, the time without the drugs makes them feel unwell (it is called the sickness) as they are experiencing various stages of withdrawal.

Current actions by addicts in America and elsewhere in the world continually seek to blame pharmaceutical companies, governments, aid providers, police and medical practitioners for their addiction and related problems.

The core, however, in my view is that there are too many

people who decide to take the easy way out of life and remain in a constant state of euphoria at the expense of others.

Having made these comments, there is no doubt that such drugs are highly addictive and can have some serious side effects, so they must be treated with caution.

On many occasions (especially after a big night out) I have thought that just taking one of these opioid tablets would make the symptoms go away and make my day better. That is where the choice comes in, and where the thought process has to be that taking addictive pain medication to get over a hangover or because I am feeling a bit down is a slippery slope and will only lead to more use and possible addiction.

The hook is that opioid drugs make you feel great, and it is hard to replicate these feelings in real life.

However, surely, when a user progresses from taking one or two tablets a day to taking 30 or 40, or crushing and snorting them, injecting or smoking the substance, there should be some realisation that things are getting out of control, and some sort of brake should be applied.

Nancy Reagan's 'Just Say No' program launched in the 1980s in the so-called 'War on Drugs' was relevant then and is relevant now.

Addicts appear to have turned the debate around to where they are the injured party and the rest of society is at fault for their predicament.

For me, the opioid drugs were brilliant, but I certainly had some issues with them. The first symptom to appear while on morphine was intense itching from inside my body, from what felt like just beneath the surface of my skin. The itching was intense and scary at the time.

When I asked the duty nurse about the symptom, she casually advised that sometimes the pain meds caused this reaction. Nobody had mentioned this to me before the meds were administered, and I was not given any advice on how to deal with the uncomfortable side effect of the drug/s.

The other symptom that surfaced was that I experienced rigours and massive night sweats a couple of days after the surgery. These were uncomfortable and required the changing of pyjamas and bedclothes each night. Again, when I inquired about these symptoms, I was advised that sometimes they occur after surgery. It would have been nice to know beforehand.

I looked this symptom up on the internet and sure enough it is quite common after surgery and usually lasts for about 10 days after it. Pethidine is found to be effective in reducing post-operative shivering.

I learnt to manage these symptoms myself through research and trial and error when I returned home from the hospital. I discovered that the chills and fevers usually occurred in the middle of the night and I needed a better regime to deal with the disruption to sleep to both myself and my wife.

I placed a spare pillow by the bed, slept on a large beach towel on top of the sheets and had spare pyjamas next to the bed.

These actions allowed me to get more rest by not having to change sheets, pillows and pyjamas as often through the night.

When you have just had major surgery and are loaded up with painkillers in the hospital and sent home, quite often these symptoms occur and you do not have access to the same pain medication as administered in the hospital.

I have found it common to be heavily medicated on release and happy to leave (due to the euphoric feelings associated with the opioid pain medication) only to find that 24 to 48 hours later, the real ordeal begins at home.

Over the last 10 years or so of my surgeries, in addition to fentanyl often replacing morphine as pain medication, tramadol has replaced oxycodone (e.g. Endone, Oxycontin, OxyNorm).

During my second partial nephrectomy in 2018, I was told I had a collapsed lung arising from the extended time lying on my side during surgery.

As a result of this complication, I had difficulty breathing and was prescribed massive doses of antibiotics to deal with the associated pneumonia that the collapsed lung had precipitated.

Combined with the surgical recovery, I could have done without this complication but I had to deal with it. A day or two out of my recovery, I was dealing with the following issues:

- Pain from the surgical procedure
- Night chills, rigours and sweats
- Collapsed lung and pneumonia
- Itchy skin
- Lack of appetite
- Catheter full and not removed when it should have been.

Apart from these issues, I was in a private room in a private hospital paying around $3,000 per night. It was the middle of summer on the Gold Coast and the air conditioning in my room was faulty so that I was sweating profusely and uncomfortable all through the day.

I decided it was time to fix these issues and asked to see the nurse in charge, advising her that:

- I needed the full catheter removed immediately
- I needed to be moved to a room where the air conditioning worked efficiently
- I needed my dressings removed as they were having

an allergic reaction to my skin. The hospital had been notified of this well in advance and details were in my patient file and on the noticeboard in my room

- I wanted off the tramadol as the drugs I was taking simply were not managing the pain. I wanted to be placed back on oxycodone immediately. I agreed to stay on the Targin but would have preferred morphine or pethidine. Even though constipation is worse with morphine and there may be some detriment to breathing, in my view it was a far better drug under the circumstances.

I told her I was well aware that the decision to limit these drugs was only based on politics related to addiction risks, and in my view the replacement drugs were ineffective in my case. I was well aware of the addiction risks with morphine and oxycodone and was able to manage these risks.

I said that if these actions did not occur reasonably quickly, I would be forced to leave the hospital and seek care at home in an air-conditioned environment where I had access to suitable painkillers and treatment.

Fortunately, my requests were agreed to, and they apologised for the lack of treatment I was receiving, although again, they told me they were understaffed and there were many people on the ward sicker than I was.

Anyone seeing a pattern here?

Tip Number 15

If you are going to be a number, be number 1.

The purpose of this book is to describe some of the things that occur outside the main game, and how I dealt with them.

Sometimes, the side effects of medications are well known to the medical fraternity but the information is not readily passed on to the patient.

Following my heart attack and stent insertion, I was prescribed a low dose of a drug named Coversyl (perindopril), commonly prescribed to help lower blood pressure.

Shortly after the heart surgery I developed a dry, irritating, persistent cough and shortness of breath which disturbed my sleep, increased fatigue and was generally annoying. The cough was not relieved by any over-the-counter medication.

At an appointment with my GP approximately four months after the heart surgery, he noticed my cough and asked when it had appeared. After a brief examination he said it was a common side effect of Coversyl. He had a discussion with my heart specialist and I was prescribed a different drug which had no further effects and the cough disappeared.

My point here is that it appears the 'Coversyl cough' is well known and symptomatic in approximately a third of people who take the drug. Just search for this phrase online and you will see what I mean. If the symptom is so prolific, why don't clinicians tell you that Coversyl patients may develop a dry cough and shortness of breath and to contact the GP or the surgeon to discuss an alternative if it happens to you?

I spoke with one heart patient who put up with the cough for nearly three years before the Coversyl cough was diagnosed. Her symptoms disappeared immediately when she was taken off the drug.

I am aware of some of the legal issues that clinicians face and the drug company lists of possible side effects that accompany every drug, and I understand why clinicians cannot list every side effect of every drug they prescribe. However, there are some very common side effects of drugs such as prednisone, Coversyl and others mentioned in this book associated with cancer treatments that in my view should be raised with the patient to save potential discomfort.

Tip Number 16

If you are prescribed drugs, conduct your own research into their common side effects and relative contraindications (possible adverse reactions with other drugs, which under certain circumstances may be necessary when the benefits outweighs the risks). If you are experiencing any of the side effects, contact your GP and/or treating specialist to discuss your concerns.

Do the research anyway, whether you are experiencing side effects or not, so that you can understand the drug, its use and possible contraindications.

Some of the basic rules that I made up and applied to my circumstances were as follows:

1. Lying in bed feeling sorry for yourself is in some cases the only option, such as on day eight or nine after chemotherapy, or after surgery that restricts movement and exercise. Under these circumstances I tried to keep mentally active by researching issues I was interested in, watching movies, reading books and generally interacting with people.

2. I tried not to dwell on the negative aspects of my circumstances and worked really hard on living day by day. This was one of the hardest things I found to do mentally, as I like to plan things and be one step ahead.

But focusing on little pleasures and small things on a daily basis can help lift your mood. Often, the treatments and recovery are over a long period and if your fitness and mental health can improve in conjunction with the medical intervention, the chances of a positive outcome are improved.

3. The positive benefits of physical exercise are well documented and should be part of your recovery plan. Recording milestones in your medical log/file will provide positive feedback when reviewed and deliver achievable goals. In my case I ran a route up a hill on a well-known seaside local track that I had trained on for over 15 years. The first time I attempted to run the hill after a chemotherapy treatment, I got about two thirds of the way and marked in my mind the spot where I stopped. Each time after that attempt I ran a little bit further, until through incremental improvement I was able to run the whole track again. During this period I had setbacks and felt fatigued, sick and depressed and could hardly get my feet moving. However, I persevered and found that just getting out of the house, going to the beach and having a walk took time out of my day, lifted my spirits, provided some form of exercise and made me generally feel better.

4. Planning and going for a simple walk, for a person not undergoing treatment, can be straightforward. For a

cancer patient mid-treatment, it can be a complex and harrowing ordeal. Some bodily functions are at times unreliable, so choose somewhere that has public facilities close by if possible. Don't overdo it and make yourself more fatigued or sick. It is a fine balance to listen to your body and know when to go and when to stop.

5. Some personal trainers are skilled in dealing with cancer patients and provide tailored exercise programs to suit your circumstances. But as with everything else, your exercise program should be checked by your treating medical specialists or your GP before you commence. I used one for a limited time then based on some of their advice, designed a program that suited me that I could do at home or on a walk or run.

6. When I wasn't hungry, I would make a fruit smoothie to give me energy. It was part of my ritual to exercise about two hours after I consumed the drink.

7. Building an exercise regime into your day provides positive goals and gets the body and mind moving. Some days I was so sick that all I could manage was to get up, have a hot shower, get dressed and then go outside and walk 10 times around the outdoor table. The fact that I did all of these actions and some exercise gave me immense satisfaction and a mental lift.

8. Look the part by putting on runners and walking shorts, a t-shirt and a hat. Nobody else needs to know that you

are not well or in recovery. It makes you feel positive and helps you blend in with everybody else, no matter how sick you are.

Tip Number 17

Living through your cancer experience takes attitude, planning, dedication and working in conjunction with your medical treatment to get the best results. Planning all the aspects of your treatment, the possible side effects, days when you can and can't exercise, and what you can and cannot achieve are all methods of controlling what you can control and dealing with as best you can the things you cannot.

Tip Number 18

Reducing fatigue and improving your mental and physical health are positive ways of contributing to the end result.

Tip Number 19

Any exercise is better than none, and although most of us when going through the process have days of despair and sickness, the achievement of small goals and improvements through increased activity levels and sleep patterns can aid recovery much better than the opposite.

I don't understand why patients undergoing cancer treatment cannot be given a straightforward information sheet that details broadly the chemicals/surgery/radiation treatment they are about to undertake and a list of possible side effects to watch out for, along with some simple tips like those in this book to alleviate the symptoms of the side effects.

However, nothing beats discussions with your treating clinicians and conducting your own research into your side effects to manage these issues quickly.

After treatment

Quite often after treatment is finished, there will be follow-up medication and/or medication to stabilise your condition and prevent future occurrences arising.

Some of the collateral damage that occurs following radical and lifesaving treatments can be distressing. In my case, the loss of taste and smell, peripheral neuropathy and some of the other symptoms remain the lesser of two evils and are insignificant compared to death or the removal of limbs or body organs that some cancer patients experience.

In some cases, the medication can be reduced or stopped entirely. I am not on any cancer-related drugs at all.

But just as with going through the various stages of cancer, from diagnosis to the end of treatment, your health, fitness and mental attitude remain in my view the key elements to work with in conjunction with your treatment regime. These help build on the success of finishing the treatment and staying above ground.

It must be recognised that after a series of events such as the cancer journey, your body has gone through huge changes and in some cases it has been poisoned, radiated, cut open and generally dealt some harsh blows.

Therefore, it is best to give your body the opportunity to recover in stages so that the outcomes achieved from the treatment are allowed to consolidate and then improve.

Some of the cancer drugs can stay in the system for long periods after they have been stopped, so exercise and drinking lots of water assist in cleansing the system and allowing the body to heal naturally.

Immediately after treatment, chemotherapy drugs generally stay in the system for about 48 hours before they are broken down by the body.

During this time, sex without a condom should be avoided and also:

- Flush the toilet twice with the lid down after each use
- If you vomit, clean up any spilt vomit and if in a bucket or other reusable receptacle, wash it out with soap and water
- Family or caregivers should wear two pairs of disposable gloves if they need to touch any of your bodily fluids
- Clothes with bodily fluids should be washed in a washing machine and not by hand
- Avoid becoming pregnant during chemotherapy.

Hopefully, steroids and anti-nausea drugs will also finish after the treatments. With radiation and surgery, the effects gradually dissipate, scars fade and rashes disappear.

If you are required to continue with medication and/or treatment, seek advice from your treating doctors about the duration of the medication/treatments and when they can be reduced or stopped if possible.

The incremental changes that occur as your body heals and your fitness increases also provide the benefits of better mental health, increased appetite, strength and mobility.

Physical exercise has so many recognised benefits, but for cancer patients it can be an escape from all of the things associated with your specific treatment.

A walk in the fresh air or even a push in a wheelchair on a nice day provides feelings hard to replicate with television, food and drugs.

Just for men, I also found that not shaving made me look untidy and even worse than I felt, so I shaved every two or three days.

However, I have also known male cancer patients who have used their recovery time to grow nice beards and moustaches, so once again it is horses for courses.

Chapter 6

How to Maximise the Effects of Treatment

Depending upon what treatment you are undergoing, there will be a recovery period relative to that treatment and your medical issues.

This recovery period generally starts after the more dramatic aspects of the treatment have been endured, such as the first few days after surgery or when a series of chemotherapy/radiation treatments has ceased.

The feelings of physical discomfort and fatigue are generally accompanied by feelings of anxiety about your future prospects and work, family and life in general. It is important not to catastrophise your feelings and become overwhelmed by the magnitude of the issues to be dealt with.

I found it incredibly difficult to apply that trite but true 'take it one day at a time' attitude because there were so many things to deal with after the invasive medical interventions ceased.

Fortunately, as difficult as it was, this one day at a time attitude helped me greatly during my recovery.

I set achievable goals and made sure that I achieved them within reasonable timeframes. This included devising and delivering appropriate rewards.

While undergoing treatment for cancer, planning is important, but it must be paced out to suit the circumstances. For example, it is pointless to worry about the next three chemotherapy treatments or upcoming surgery if you are still suffering the effects of the last treatment. You need to wait to see what the outcomes are and whether that treatment is working or another treatment may be prescribed.

Not all treatments are successful and often, changes are made to medication or surgery to suit the changed circumstances. Unfortunately, the cancer patient has to deal with these changes as they arise and be able to have a positive and flexible mindset to accommodate the changes.

Not all news is good news. Depending upon the seriousness of the condition, quite often a patient has to hear confronting and distressing news concerning their condition, medication, treatment or all of these matters combined.

Sometimes treatments don't work, other methods must be attempted, more treatments or surgery must be undertaken and timeframes must be altered.

This is where my attitude of splitting what I could deal with and what I could not became a way of life while undergoing the various treatments.

When I took the medication, I tried to stay as positive as possible. I looked after my health and mindset and stayed focused on each step. Then I would eventually improve incrementally until things got better.

This is easy to say but difficult to carry out when you are in the middle of a chemotherapy/surgery cycle and as sick as can be possibly imagined.

It is also a real and present possibility that the treatments will not be successful, and your lifespan is shortened, but dwelling on this possibility is counterproductive.

One criticism I have of some medical professionals is the attitude that the patient deserves to be told the absolute truth about their condition and their possible time left to live. This is usually after all viable options have been explored and there is no hope of recovery or cure, with palliative care and certain death the only outcomes.

I have seen and spoken in depth with cancer patients who have been told that they have no hope and limited time to live.

There are a number of factors which seem to be prevalent under these circumstances, which include:

- Every patient, disease and reaction to drugs and treatment is closely linked to their family history and race, age, mental health, physical and biological constitution, attitude, support structures, finances, treating professionals and access to treatment facilities
- There are major breakthroughs in medicine, technology and science almost daily that may provide new and/or more successful treatments
- Most human beings strive to stay alive, and the body can produce amazing results under the direst of circumstances
- Death is inevitable, and each person faces their immortality in different ways, but the bottom line is we will all die at some stage, and a perceived premature death through cancer is actually not a premature death it is just death, the same as death through accident or misadventure
- Common threads amongst human beings such as aspiration, the pursuit of happiness, the will to live and the survival instinct can be trashed when hope is removed.

Imagine telling soldiers in battle that the war was lost, their efforts were in vain, the position was hopeless, but their orders were to attack the enemy position in front of them with the outcome that they would all be killed.

Hardly the way to motivate people.

In my experience, the same principle applies to how some medical professionals deliver the news that the patient's condition is terminal, there is no hope of a cure and, given an estimated timeframe, they should get ready for the end of life.

While in many cases this information is factually correct, the timeframes depend on many variables, as indicated above. Although the outcome may be sooner or later than the indicated timeframe, the absence of hope is soul-destroying and finite.

For these reasons, I have generally ascribed to my own view of life. Faced with possible death on many occasions over the last 10 years, I have defied the odds and continue to be positive and physically present every day of my life.

Even faced with the inevitability of imminent death, I would wring out the last drops of fun and get the maximum bang for my buck while my time on earth remained.

All the things that are deemed 'bad' would be back on the table depending upon my physical capabilities, such as cigarettes, eating and drinking anything I felt like with no regard for my health, and physical pursuits such as skydiving and swimming with great white sharks.

My experience was that lying in bed contemplating the future when diagnosed with cancer and about to start or in the middle of treatment was the least healthy option for me.

On the days in the middle of my chemotherapy treatments when my prognosis was dire and the first treatment had not been successful, I had the view that anything I did that made me happy was a good thing, and if I died doing something I wanted to do, or after doing it, then so be it.

Death is an inevitable part of life, and for some people so is illness and despair, but there is always hope. Hope of a new cure, hope that a miracle occurs, hope that things improve and you live a few more months or years than predicted.

Every minute of extra time on earth is valuable and if pain management is done correctly the last few days, hours and minutes should be cherished.

Recently, my wife's father suffered a serious stroke and was found unconscious in his home about five hours' travel away from us. His doctor contacted us and said that her father was in hospital and unlikely to survive for more than 24 hours, so not to worry about driving there to see him.

We ignored this advice, drove to the hospital and went to see him the next day. We were told that due to the severity of the stroke, he had been left paralysed and was unable to speak. They also told us (while we were in the room with the patient who was conscious and aware at the time) that he was in palliative care and would not be given food or water but would be kept sedated until his eventual death.

The problem we had with this was that he clearly recognised his daughter who was able to comfort and speak to him. He communicated through grunts and movements but was clearly aware, agitated, anxious and distressed.

I said this to the nurse and asked how much sedation was being administered. She said 5 mg of Diazepam, four-hourly.

The patient was struggling to swallow, had no liquid, obviously had a parched throat and his breathing was laboured and stertorous.

We were not satisfied with this treatment plan, and in very clear terms I told the nurse that my father in-law was obviously distressed and was not being cared for in a humane way. We wanted the treatment improved and wanted to speak with the doctor.

I told her that in my view such a small dose of Diazepam was useless, and was obviously not controlling the pain or the symptoms, and if they did not remedy the situation and improve his treatment then I would look at what action we would need to take to fix the issues.

The doctor contacted us by phone later that night, and in no uncertain terms we told him what we thought about the way our family member was being treated. We said that we expected the treatment to be drastically improved, and we would not be leaving until the matter had been resolved or he succumbed to his medical condition.

The next day we went to the hospital to see him and although the nurses were not very happy to see us, there was a marked difference in his condition.

A senior nurse came into the ward and advised us that after speaking to the doctor, the treatment had been revised and he had been given an increased dosage of anti-anxiety drugs, antispasmodic drugs so that he could swallow and some water for his parched throat.

There was a significant difference in his attitude. There were no jerky movements, no drool and no obvious signs of distress like we had seen the day before. He clearly recognised us, and our presence calmed him further.

I was still not happy and asked the nurse why this had not been done before, and what an ignominious, lonely and pathetic death he would have suffered if we had followed the doctor's advice and not come to see him.

I said that we would stay with him until he died and make sure he received appropriate and caring treatment.

He lasted for another four days after these events and died a relatively peaceful death.

Apart from it being my wife's father, this was a traumatic and eye-opening incident for us because we saw that the euthanasia debate with all of its complexities remains apparent in hospitals today. This is because of the relative inaction patients in palliative care may experience in their treatment, on occasion bordering on cruel and inhumane.

In my mind it defies belief that on the one hand they advised us he was in palliative care and would not last more than 24 hours and not to bother to go and see him. On the other hand, when we disregarded this advice, we found that he was being literally starved to death with minimum pain relief and they were just waiting for him to die in his bed.

I am still angry about what we went through to improve his final few days, and it affected us so deeply that my wife and I made formal advance health directives to clearly stipulate our wishes in relation to our specific medical treatment if placed in a similar position.

It defies description why the medical staff administered such a low dose of pain/anxiety medication to an obviously suffering man.

The chances of him becoming addicted to morphine or oxycodone in his state and stage of life were so remote that they should not have been considered, and when I raised this with the doctor, I called it for the bullshit it was.

The reason I retell this story in my book is the same reason as the inclusion of the other events, to show that despite the best intentions of medical staff, hospitals, doctors or anyone else involved in your treatment, sometimes things go bad. When they do, you need to step on it straightaway and seek a resolution or positive changes.

During my treatments, rewards were not always material things, but sometimes I would have a walk along the beach and a nice lunch with family after a particularly harrowing period or procedure. Other times I would indulge in a splash of retail therapy and buy myself something I liked just because I deserved it.

I am a strong believer in reminders and positive reinforcement, and my particular idiosyncrasy is the purchase of watches to remind me of specific events or achievements. This goes all the way back to my time in the oil industry when I smoked and drank heavily.

When my first child, our daughter, was born my wife and I both stopped smoking by going cold turkey and I have not smoked since in over 30 years.

At the time, quitting smoking was very difficult as I had smoked for about 18 years and in my job at the time I was under massive stress.

My role then was as the Senior Industrial Relations Adviser for Esso Australia. I had responsibility for industrial relations for the Bass Strait oilfield operations, which at the time was the largest economical project in the Southern Hemisphere. It contributed 10% of Australia's GDP and was one of the most volatile industrial and union environments in the world.

My job was critically assessed as one of the most difficult in its field in the world at the time and it certainly lived up to its reputation.

I was a chain smoker, smoking anywhere from 40 to 100 cigarettes a day, every day. When I quit, I went to the best jewellery store in town and picked out a nice moderately expensive wristwatch and placed it on lay-by.

I calculated at the time my monthly expenditure on cigarettes and committed this amount to the purchase and lay-by payment plan.

Every time I thought about having a cigarette, I thought about my nice new watch and when I could get it, concentrating on that goal and not my nicotine cravings.

I also went to a naturopath and followed a cleansing diet for a few weeks to aid the process, but after two weeks of black pumpernickel bread, lettuce leaves and water I decided that if this was living then I wanted out, and reverted to food that was healthy but had some substance and taste.

I have continued this watch purchase method throughout my life and currently have over 30 nice watches. Each one of them reminds me of a milestone event so that when I am wearing one, I am reminded of a positive time in my life or an achievement.

I do not treat this ritual lightly and reserve it for occasions like the end of chemotherapy treatments, achieving a significant training or sporting goal or an event that is important in my life or family.

I recently bought a watch to commemorate the death of a close friend and mentor so that I would be reminded of our friendship and the influence he'd had on my life and career.

I only wear this watch in court or during legal issues as he was an expert in the field, and we worked together for many years.

It is not so much the acquisition or wearing of the watches that works for me, it is the positive reinforcement and reminders of past achievements and life milestones that constantly make me feel good.

During some consultations where I have received bad news or am advised that I require further treatment, I will look at the watch I am wearing (carefully chosen to suit the event) and remember what I have been through before and how successful I have been in managing the issues I faced at that time, or I might remember celebrating a family or lifestyle event which made me very happy.

These triggers are important to manage the myriad of thoughts that must be managed going forward when your recovery commences.

This period is in my view a true representation of the word 'holistic'. In order to get the best outcome and maximise your chances of survival, your whole environment must be involved.

I identified early on in my treatments that if I let depression and anxiety enter the equation then my chances of recovery would be dramatically reduced.

I chose to look upon my early diagnosis as a bonus and the

medical treatments as my lifesavers rather than something to be endured.

I did as much research as I could on the side effects of the treatments and medicines I was taking and tried to tailor my lifestyle to suit what complemented them best.

I found this period straight after the treatments/surgery to be the hardest, simply because the good drugs administered in the hospital have usually been stopped. Once home, you are faced with the after-effects of the treatments and all the ongoing management issues that people not having these problems do not have to face.

Simple things like planning your day are hugely important. For example, if you are unable to move for a period of weeks following surgery or are incapacitated for some other reason, it is vital to do something with your time other than lying in bed feeling sorry for yourself.

This is the time when depression can kick in, and keeping your mind active and positive can ward off these symptoms.

However, it must be recognised that grief and feelings of sadness cannot be removed from the equation. Anyone suffering from cancer or any other life-threatening disease is in my view entitled to have these feelings and experience times when a good cry is the best option.

The trick is to move on quickly and look for the positives that exist in your life and build on them.

Tip Number 20

Enjoy the little things in life, for one day you'll look back and realise they were the big things.

Everybody's view about what to do in recovery may be different but for me, keeping motivated and mentally active was crucial.

I have written and published eight guides on human resources, industrial relations and employee relations dealing with the technical application of laws and regulatory frameworks to drugs and alcohol in the workplace and stress management. These were sold online through a marketing/publishing business, and I used my recovery time when I was unable to move to work on these products.

I reread them all, made changes, updated technical and legal details and increased the library by writing a whole new product aimed at increasing the market and improving the products in general.

I also maintained client contact and was able to provide advice and work on contracts, policies and general business from my bed.

My only restriction was I was unable to physically attend meetings/hearings for a while, so I referred these matters to others so that my clients had the services they required.

This was my only restriction because in today's world, communication is available at so many levels. I used online messaging, FaceTime, email and messaging to stay in contact with my clients and to provide them with the services they needed.

These activities not only provided an income stream, but they kept me focused and active even though I was bedbound at times and feeling pretty rough.

The advantages were that I chose the work I accepted based on my capabilities and limitations, I was able to rest between work assignments, I did not jeopardise my recovery by being overactive and I felt connected with the world.

I planned my day carefully and made sure that I had the following items close by:

1. Laptop and stable table
2. Smartphone and charger
3. Notebook and pen
4. Drink of water next to bed
5. My required medication
6. Extendable arm to reach items when required
7. Books to read
8. Television with streaming services on bedroom wall.

If you are not able to work from home in your own business like I did, and you are employed externally, ask your employer about their work from home options/policies and see if you can maintain some part of your job while in your recovery period.

If you are not employed, there is a multitude of options to stop boredom and depression from setting in such as:

1. Play online games
2. FaceTime friends and family
3. Commence an online study course
4. Watch movies and TV
5. Plan your activities step by step to coincide with your recovery
6. Set goals and devise appropriate rewards.

There are also days when it is OK just to lie in bed and suffer. I had many days like this especially on days eight or nine after chemotherapy. Lying in bed and dribbling were all I was capable of. When such days occur, deal with them and know that the next day will be better.

Tip Number 21

It is part of recovery to have days of pain or fatigue or sickness. This is part of the healing process and should be embraced for what it is. It is not the end of the world.

In order to maximise the benefits of whatever treatment you have undergone it is important to give yourself the best shot at obtaining the best possible results. This is where choices come in to play.

If you finish treatment and go on a diet of junk food and fizzy drinks combined with a sedentary lifestyle, lying around all day feeling depressed, taking large doses of painkillers, having little or no contact with friends, family and the outside world, you can expect your recovery to be slow and success is not guaranteed.

I am not saying don't do this, but I am saying that these are personal choices and you can choose good ones or bad ones. The choices are yours.

Tip Number 22

Battling cancer is a life or death fight and should be treated as such. The battle won't be won unless the good fight is fought.

Many of the tests, medication and invasive procedures that form part of cancer treatments have never been experienced before by the body and are quite unique.

Chemotherapy for example is a chemical used to destroy

cancer cells in the body so they can be replaced by new cancer-free cells.

Chemotherapy was discovered between 1943 and 1946 during World War 2, where it was found that soldiers exposed to mustard gas had reduced white blood cell counts.

Mustard gas reacts quickly with water in the airways where it forms hydrochloric acid and acts to swell and block tissue in the lungs, causing suffocation.

Soldiers subjected to large doses of mustard gas died from blistering of the lungs and throat.

It is estimated that there were 1.3 million casualties and 90,000 deaths in World War 1 from the use of mustard gas.

Researchers then used this information to see if the mustard gas chemicals could be used against rapidly growing cancer cells. Trials were conducted on non-Hodgkin lymphoma using a less volatile form of the mustard gas called mustine (nitrogen mustard).

This commenced the use of cytotoxic drugs in treating cancers and was followed by discoveries using folic acid and vinka alkaloids extracted from vinca rosea, which were beneficial in certain leukaemia cancer treatments. These resulted in vinca alkaloids such as vinblastine and vincristine to treat Hodgkin's disease and leukaemia.

Such a toxic and deadly chemical being used to treat cancer is a revelation in itself. It reinforces my point that these chemicals are something the body has never experienced before and should be treated accordingly.

What I mean by this is that a person's experiences prior to chemotherapy treatment are only based on the illnesses and medications they have been exposed to over their life up until the start of the chemotherapy.

Chemotherapy drugs can, and do, cause some feelings, sensations and after-effects that are beyond most people's normal experiences and imagination.

It is obviously not the same as a mustard gas attack, but neither is it like taking aspirin for a headache. Some discomfort must be expected.

If doctors provide you with anti-nausea drugs or any other medication that can help alleviate some of the symptoms of the treatment, then my advice is to take them while you can.

It becomes a real balancing act to manage all your personal matters, including how you cope with the treatment, how you relate to family and friends, how you manage finances and long- and short-term goals.

Planning too far ahead can be distressing at times because sometimes life and other things get in the way of plans, so expectations need to be practical and flexible.

Once the treatment is concluded and the medical practitioners have done as much as they can do for now, there is a period of reflection and assessment of what has happened during your treatment. What are the after-effects, what does your future hold, are there follow-up treatments, what can you do to improve your outcomes?

Hopefully, reading this book will help you consider making choices that are in your best interests and aid your recovery while improving your future prospects.

Chapter 7

Coping Mechanisms Pre- and Post-treatment

By reading this book, I know you are alive and already in front of the game. Staying alive and retaining your sanity through the cancer journey is the real challenge.

Once the trauma of the diagnosis and the knowledge that your life is about to change dramatically have been digested and dealt with, you have to determine the way that you intend to approach your challenges and forge ahead.

Stress, anxiety and depression can be debilitating in their own right and in this chapter, I explain the tools that I used to get me through the process. These give you some options to consider.

My method immediately following my original cancer diagnosis was not to fall victim to stress, anxiety and depression, and to give my brain and body the best possible chance at overcoming the disease and surviving the treatments.

While a certain level of stress is necessary to avoid boredom, high levels of stress over a sustained period can damage your health. In the absence of the ability to run away or to physically attack (fight or flight), the individual often responds in one or a number of the following ways:

BODY'S REACTION TO STRESS	RESPONSE TO STRESS			
	Physical	Behavioural	Thinking	Emotions
• Adrenaline increases • Increased heart rate • Higher blood pressure • Dilated pupils • Hands cold and clammy • Perspiration • Numb to pain • Goose bumps	• Headaches • Back pain • Fatigue • Upset stomach/ ulcers • Digestive disorders • Muscle tension • Sexual dysfunction • Sweating • Back pain • Irregular heart rate • Frequent colds • Skin problems • Insomnia • Fatigue	• Eat poorly • Excessive smoking • Abuse drugs or alcohol • Drive or act recklessly • Accident-prone • Poor communication • Extreme anger	• Poor concentration • Forgetfulness • Learning difficulties • Speech problems • Obsessive negative thoughts	• Anxiety • Depression • Sadness • Anger • Impatience • Irritability • Feeling of helplessness

Many of the physiological and emotional changes listed in the table are linked. When you look at these reactions to stress, why would you want to exacerbate your symptoms and add to your cancer issues by bringing in more damaging and potentially dangerous symptoms? Especially when you can control these symptoms and use stress reduction techniques to assist your healing processes and achieve the best possible outcome.

For example, those in a state of anxiety will have a rise in heart rate, and those suffering from tension and depression may have bouts of insomnia. Compound these symptoms with the drug-related side effects of some of the cancer medication and a bad situation can quickly become a drastic situation.

While the symptoms in isolation may or may not show stress, where several occur it is likely that stress is having an effect.

If prolonged, this effect can adversely affect your ability to react positively to medication and treatment and your recovery in both the long and short term.

While symptoms of stress vary for each person, they may include:

- Psychological and emotional
  › Denial
  › Anxiety and fear
  › Worry about safety of self and others
  › Anger

- › Irritability
- › Restlessness
- › Sadness, grief, depression, moodiness
- › Distressing dreams
- › Feeling overwhelmed, hopeless
- › Feeling isolated, lost, abandoned
- › Apathy
- Cognitive
  - › Memory problems
  - › Disorientation
  - › Confusion
  - › Slowness of thinking and comprehension
  - › Difficulty calculating, setting priorities, making decisions
  - › Poor concentration
  - › Limited attention span
  - › Loss of objectivity
  - › Dwelling on negative aspects of diagnosis/treatment
  - › Blaming
- Behavioural
  - › Change in activity
  - › Decreased efficiency and effectiveness
  - › Difficulty communicating
  - › Increased sense of humour
  - › Outbursts of anger, frequent arguments
  - › Inability to rest or calm down

- › Change in eating habits
- › Change in sleeping patterns
- › Change in patterns of intimacy, sexuality
- › Change in job performance (if still working during treatment)
- › Periods of crying
- › Increased use of alcohol, tobacco or other drugs
- › Social withdrawal, silence
- › Vigilance about safety or environment
- › Avoidance of activities or places that trigger memories
- › Proneness to accidents
- Physical
  - › Increased heartbeat, respiration
  - › Increased blood pressure
  - › Upset stomach, nausea, diarrhoea
  - › Change in appetite, weight loss or gain
  - › Sweating or chills
  - › Tremors (hands, lips)
  - › Muscle twitching
  - › 'Muffled' hearing
  - › Tunnel vision
  - › Feeling uncoordinated
  - › Headaches
  - › Soreness in muscles
  - › Lower back pain
  - › Feeling a 'lump in the throat'

> › Exaggerated startle reaction
> › Fatigue
> › Menstrual cycle changes
> › Change in sexual desire
> › Decreased resistance to infection
> › Flare-up of allergies and arthritis
> › Hair loss.

However, not all stress is bad. A moderate amount of stress may actually improve your ability to perform tasks. Nevertheless, people faced with a diagnosis of cancer or serious and invasive medical procedures and medicines may experience heightened levels of stress, which can adversely affect their ability to navigate the cancer journey.

There are two main types of stress that people experience:

1. **Eustress**

   The stress that facilitates your efforts (good stress).

2. **Distress**

   The stress that has a negative impact on your ability to function or cope with certain situations.

The difficulty is that there are no clear definitions for what the impact can be, as each person experiences stress differently.

Some people rarely experience high levels of stress in their lives, while others experience it regularly. Also, some are more able to cope with stress levels than others.

Stress reduction strategies

Dr Harold Minden identified four main approaches to reducing stress:

- Symptom reduction strategies
- Problem-solving strategies
- Adaptation strategies
- Prevention strategies.

Symptom reduction strategies

- Reducing physical tension by taking deep breaths, calming self through meditation, walking mindfully.
- Using time off for exercise, reading, listening to music, taking a bath, talking to family or having a special meal to recharge batteries.
- Talking about emotions and reactions with family, friends or co-workers at appropriate times.
- Cognitive strategies (e.g. constructive self-talk, restructuring distortions).
- Relaxation techniques (e.g. yoga, meditation, guided imagery).
- Pacing self between low and high stress activities and between performing activities both alone and with support.

Some of the more common symptom reduction strategies include:

- Acupuncture
- Aromatherapy
- Exercise
- Religion
- Sex
- Rocking
- Swedish massage
- Shiatsu
- Worry beads
- Stress balls
- Diet
- Music
- Biofeedback
- Pets.

Problem-solving strategies

Instead of helping to reduce the symptoms of stress, problem-solving strategies serve to remove or cut off the source of stress.

This involves identifying various sources of stress and thinking about the way the problem might be solved.

For stressors that can be removed, problem-solving strategies can have a major impact on your stress levels.

This can be as simple as understanding your treatments and possible side effects, such as nausea during chemotherapy infusions; arranging a support person to go with you; not eating beforehand; talking to your doctor about anti-nausea medication; meditating; arranging for suitable transport home after the treatment; any other practical step that will help you get through the treatment.

Taking these steps can give you reassurance that you have some control over your concerns. Even if the worst happens, you know you have taken as many steps as possible to deal with them.

Applying this planning and strategic approach ties in with my initial advice to treat the events as a triathlon with many segments, beginning with the preparation and training and going all the way through to the end of the event and recovery.

Adaptation strategies

Sometimes, we simply cannot change a stressful situation. In these circumstances, it is important to find a way to adapt to the unchanging reality you face. This may mean making lifestyle-based decisions to either accept the challenges you face by adapting, or mapping out a practical strategy and timetable to move towards change that suits your current circumstances and future needs.

Prevention strategies

Some events are cyclical and cause stress each time they come around, so it is important to recognise these triggers and plan to deal with them in the most effective manner. An example of these are chemotherapy infusions or regular radiation treatments. Look for ways to effectively manage these stressors so that they have a lesser impact the next time around. Remember that each time you go through a treatment, surgery or radiation event, you are one step closer to the end of the treatment when your body can start to heal, hopefully minus the cancer.

Eliminating stress from your environment

If your living and working environments are badly organised, they can be a major source of stress. If your environment is well organised and pleasant, it can help to reduce stress and increase productivity. Remember though that while it may be important for people under stress to have a calm environment, others may enjoy the raised levels of arousal associated with the 'buzz' of a busy and vibrant environment.

Tip Number 23

Self-talk is important, so removing negative thoughts and catastrophising is something that you and only you can control. This thought alone becomes a powerful tool.

You can choose to be angry and you can choose to be sad.

You can also choose to be happy and positive.

A simple strategy that can benefit anybody is to trick your brain into a better place.

One of these tricks is to smile and tell yourself that things are good, and you are happy when faced with bad news, pain or feelings of apprehension and anxiety.

By looking at what you are telling yourself, looking at your thinking, at your irrational beliefs and self-defeating attitudes, you can change them to preferences instead of absolute musts.

You can then experience 'normal' stressful reactions.

In other words, you can create healthy tension and thoughts instead of unhealthy distress.

People are disturbed not by things, but their view of things
—Epictetus (Ancient Greek Stoic philosopher)

In my experience, stress reduction strategies and exercises, meditation breathing techniques and positive thinking combined with physical and mental exercise were the best possible aids to complement the medication, surgery and treatments I have had over the last 10 years.

These powerful tools when combined with the various medical interventions gave me the best outcome possible.

It is possible to prolong life and quality of life using these techniques if they are applied diligently and practically.

Another very common but effective stress reduction strategy that has been shown to produce good results, especially when practised over a long period, is the 4-7-8 breathing technique.

In this simple exercise, you breathe in through the nose for a count of four seconds, hold your breath for seven seconds and then exhale through your mouth for eight seconds.

The exercise is particularly effective for going to sleep at night. Also, practised regularly, it acts as a guided form of breathing control that calms the body and mind similar to meditation.

The beauty of these techniques is that they can be designed, tailored and implemented by individuals to suit their personal circumstances. If snake handling while singing hymns or meditating on top of a mountain in Peru works for you, then do it and do it well.

Chapter 8

How to Deal with Family and Supporters

It is not unusual for cancer patients to struggle with dealing with the outside world, friends, family and acquaintances.

For both men and women, some of the physical changes can be profound. The loss of hair, changes in general appearance and weight fluctuations accompanied by symptoms of depression, anxiety and drug-induced idiosyncrasies can be difficult to manage for the patients as well as others.

Even the task of telling friends and family that you have been diagnosed with a life-threatening illness can be difficult.

Although cancer treatments are generally more effective than they used to be, there are still some cancers that have lower survival rates. The treatments or limitations of treatments available are based on the type and location of the cancer. This makes telling people what to expect in your case extremely difficult. Often, you don't know with any certainty yourself.

Despite the best knowledge available, factors affecting outcomes include:

- Age
- Stage of cancer
- General health, including the existence of other medical conditions
- Location of cancer/s
- Treatments available
- Gender
- Mental health and attitude.

Any or all of these factors may be different for every individual, so a general cancer survival estimation may vary widely. Many patients opt simply for big picture statistics rather than seeking definite timelines, which in some cases can become self-fulfilling prophecies.

I found that it was enough information to advise family and friends I was undergoing treatment for cancer, that it would take some time and involve some fairly drastic medication, and it would hopefully treat my cancer but not cure it.

Obviously, for my closest family members and some close friends, I gave a more detailed description and updated them as required.

I also found that most people are uncomfortable when hearing this information, and they are unsure of what to say in return.

Quite often I have heard from cancer patients who are facing possible terminal illness that people say things like, 'you'll be OK', 'hope you get better' or other platitudes that do not suit their circumstances. While well-meaning, these vapid statements can be hurtful and distressing.

My favourite response to cancer patients is, 'I hope that things can be as good as they can be for you.'

I have also found that telling people the detailed truth about my condition made most people a bit squeamish and was too much information for them.

People were genuinely interested in timelines, treatment options and chances of success or failure but they had enough problems of their own to not want to be availed of every tiny detail. What's more, talking about your illness and treatments to other people can become boring for them.

Apart from these reasons, some of the events that occur during treatments are very personal and full disclosure is not warranted unless speaking with medical staff.

The truth, in my view, is always the best starting point. When you tell people that you have a serious disease but that you are undergoing treatment that has some chance of success, their response usually determines the depth of the conversation that follows.

Chapter 9

Just Do It

Surviving cancer and its associated treatments, processes and outcomes is no picnic. It requires a holistic approach that in my view is generally not understood or adequately coordinated by medical practitioners and supporting staff.

The reason for my criticism is that cancer treatment from diagnosis to post-treatment recovery affects all the following components of your life and environment:

1. Mental health
2. Physical health
3. Family and relationships
4. Finances
5. Medicine
6. Treatments
7. Doctors
8. Specialists

9. Hospitals and testing facilities
10. Environment and longevity.

All of these contain a multitude of systems, circumstances and complications that need to be managed and dealt with, essentially by the patient.

It is well documented in medical research material that certain drugs have an increased negative effect on a person's behaviour and attitude.

I have mentioned in previous chapters the effects some of these drugs had on me during my treatments and how I dealt with them. It was not easy.

Some researchers have linked the use of certain drugs, including statins, to changes in behaviour causing or contributing to road rage, pathological gambling and complicated acts of fraud and the shaping of social relationships.

Drugs as innocuous as paracetamol, antihistamines, statins, asthma medications and antidepressants have been attributed to feelings of anger, restlessness, diminished empathy and increased neurotic activity and thoughts.

Alcohol, marijuana and benzodiazepines may lead to depression, anxiety and social issues, and drugs such as Ritalin and cocaine may make a person manic.

If even a portion of this research is correct and you combine some of these drugs with chemotherapy drugs and the associated mental health issues of patients undergoing treatment and facing possible death, it is an explosive cocktail and a potential recipe for disaster.

My experience has been that treating a patient holistically by taking all these factors into account is infrequent, and I certainly have never been part of such a process.

What I have found is that each treatment, doctor, specialist or healthcare worker is focused on their contribution to your treatment/care. They usually carry out their duties to the best of their capabilities and then pass you on to the next phase of your treatment and/or recovery.

All the research conducted while writing this book pointed to one very clear conclusion from the medical fraternity: that early diagnosis is key to any condition, but especially with cancer.

Men are notorious for ignoring the symptoms of prostate cancer, and the failure to address it early can be catastrophic. One case that was brought to my attention was a middle-aged man diagnosed with early prostate cancer, who refused treatment on the grounds that his sex life at his age was more important than dealing with the prostate cancer.

He pursued alternative therapies and continued with a vigorous sex life until the symptoms of the prostate cancer became life threatening.

By then, the cancer had spread throughout his body to his bones and was untreatable.

He died a slow and agonising death in a fog of pain medication.

The doctor who discussed this case with me was clear that the early diagnosis and range of treatment options available at the time could have easily prevented this outcome.

Early presentation and diagnosis are also helpful if you are treated in the public health system, because it may take months to see a specialist and commence treatments. Meantime, the progression of a cancerous condition may be exacerbated.

One good example was the peripheral neuropathy I suffered during the chemotherapy treatments which left me with no feeling in the tips of my fingers, toes and bottoms of my feet as well as tingling and nerve pain at night.

When I advised medical practitioners of this side effect, I received sympathy and advice that it was a known possible side effect of the treatment. I was never given any advice on how to deal with it and to this day, I have to continually manage the issue.

My main point here and the essence of this chapter and the book in general is that things in life do not generally go as planned. Life can be tough and, in my opinion, we need to take responsibility for our own actions and outcomes that we can influence.

Strap yourself in for the next bit: my view on how to

overcome some of the hurdles that cancer and life can throw at you.

Tip Number 24

Don't blame society, climate change, the government or bad luck for your circumstances. If you have cancer, deal with it and give it your best shot. It will either work or it won't.

Too often, people blame other things and people for circumstances that they themselves could control. If you want to eat fast food all day, consume large amounts of soft drinks and not exercise, don't blame the manufacturers of the products for your condition. Don't expect to be healthy and breeze through cancer treatments if you continue bad and unhealthy habits.

Don't blame pharmaceutical companies, society or others for drugs and temptations that you choose to use and abuse.

My attitude to my cancer diagnosis and the associated treatments and challenges I faced was to 'just do it'. I realise that this phrase is used by Nike in their advertising campaigns, but I just concentrated on the message in the words and the actions I associated with them.

It is no good procrastinating or catastrophising, both of

which deliver poor results and lead to other conditions such as anxiety and depression.

My attitude was that I would give it my best shot and if that was not good enough, then I would have had a go and had fun along the way.

I love the saying 'it is what it is' because although trite, the statement is philosophically powerful. It emphasises that if something exists then it exists, and how you deal with it is entirely up to you.

I found that after a few blood tests, needles and insertions of too many foreign objects, the best approach was to ask what needed to be done and then to tell the person performing the task, "Just do it."

I also applied my time travel trick and focused on somewhere I was going to be in the near future when the procedure would be only a memory.

At every appointment, hospital visit, procedure or event associated with my illness and treatment, I carried a token or meditation stone. Nobody has ever noticed that I carry one in my palm during these times (obviously not during surgery). What these tokens or meditation aids do is remind me to stay calm, focus on my breathing, listen intently and not focus on pain, discomfort or anxiety.

When I go to a nice beach or other calm, relaxing place in my travels, I collect stones about the size of the top of an average thumb. The stones must be smooth and easily fit into the space between my thumb and forefinger or my palm.

I might collect five or 10 stones or shells from one location and store them at home.

With particularly pretty stones, I hold them in my palm and face the sea or the best view. Then I imprint in my mind the location, the feelings of joy, calm and peace that I'm experiencing at the time.

This imprinting process works with anything that is portable and comfortable and that reminds you of a positive experience. I use the imprinted stones and items to bring me peace and tranquillity.

They are not good luck charms; they are reminders of positive times and thoughts. I have some concern over the use of good luck charms as if one of them is lost, this can often be seen as bad luck or a bad omen and can make people quite anxious.

Obviously, the stones are free so if you lose them, it doesn't matter as there are plenty more.

On occasion I have been caught without one of my stones when facing an appointment or procedure. Then, I simply take a small item that reminds me of something other than the medical procedure. This can be anything from the vehicle you travelled in, to a piece of clothing, a pen or even a stone you pick up from the street.

I just then close my eyes and go to where I am remined of by the object.

I cannot emphasise enough the power of meditation and mind control when undergoing painful/invasive and/or distressing medical procedures or even discussions.

If you are interested and wish to explore this line of relaxation further, my advice is to look at what the Buddhist monks are able to achieve through their meditative states. You can also look into Gregorian chants. I have several different chants on my phone that I listen to when I need some serious and deep meditation, usually associated with pain and discomfort. I find the Gregorian chants the most intense and save these for particularly difficult circumstances.

It is amazing to experience the ability to turn the mind away from pain using these techniques by focusing on anything but the pain and not acknowledging pain, anxiety and discomfort.

Of course, it does not go away. However, if you focus on the pain, or the procedure, or the time, or the potential negative outcomes, if you let the pain take control of your thoughts, it is much harder to undergo the procedure and successfully manage your recovery.

In my everyday life, each time I feel pain I practise ignoring it, no matter what or where.

My favourite test is when I stub or knock my little toe on something. Instead of shouting, swearing or crying,

I consciously say inwardly, "Wow, this is another test for me to manage my pain reactions and prepare for future procedures."

I then totally ignore the sharp stabbing pain and walk away to focus on something else until I forget it.

Another good test is to go swimming and never test the temperature of the water; just dive in and deal with the consequences.

You don't see triathletes lining up for a swim at the start of the race all gingerly walking to the water's edge and dipping their toes in to test the temperature of the water. This is because they are used to training in water of all temperatures. The task is the swim, not whinging about how cold the water is. They are only focused on entering the water and commencing the race. Their minds and bodies have become conditioned to this as a normal temperature change and the body is ready to race.

This is easier than you think but you must practise it before you achieve results.

Clinical psychologists often refer to this type of thought process as controlled response therapy or cognitive behavioural therapy, abbreviated to CRT or CBT. It is used for pain management. It is also very effective in tinnitus sufferers, helping them to treat tinnitus as a background noise or feeling, rather than concentrating on the pain or on the tinnitus.

I have successfully applied these techniques to pain management with, in my view, spectacular results.

Tip Number 25

Imprint some items that remind you of pleasant places and take them with you for all treatments/procedures and medical appointments.

Chapter 10

What Next?

Life on a day-to-day basis can be confronting in many ways, but for a cancer patient, once the treatments have stopped, your view of life can sometimes be dramatically altered either positively or negatively by your experiences.

Tip Number 26

The choice of how you view the future is yours and yours alone.

Depending on whether you are at the start of your journey, have recently received the diagnosis or are at the end of your treatment and all options have been exhausted, whether successful or not, attitude and self-talk can be your greatest allies.

The sad truth is that regardless of your circumstances

there will be issues that are beyond your control or that you will have to confront, including hard decisions on treatment, medications, options and care.

I found a certain element of peace in being able to confront issues as they arose. It gave me confidence knowing that I had done as much as I could to maximise my outcomes and attitude by maintaining good mental and physical strengths.

Celebrating successes and dealing with setbacks gave me things to think about and plan for. It stopped me from being sucked into the morass of treatment, hospitals, doctors and medicine, which must be endured but does not have to become the whole focus of life.

Being miserable or happy are choices that are under your control. Your attitude can also influence your family or carers and the environment you survive in.

If you are inactive, morose and seeking pity constantly, then that is probably what you will receive in return.

People you interact with are less likely to visit and comfort you if they see a person who has given up or can only concentrate on the negativity of their circumstances.

One of my close friends used to text me every morning when he woke up, asking, Are you still breathing? while I was undergoing some of my treatments. He would also text me at random times, reminding me of how many friends I had and how we should be getting back to golf and long lunches soon.

Those short text messages were a constant reminder that I did have a life outside of the hospital ward and I had things to look forward to.

My replies to my friend's and others' texts were usually humorous and showed them that I was still in the fight.

This certainly does not mean that you cannot at times be sad, resentful or feel sorry for yourself. In my experience, the best path is to ride the roller-coaster of emotions and accept that there will be times when you are at the bottom of the hill.

From the bottom of the hill, my advice is to look up and start the climb back to the top, noting the scenery along the way.

I treated cancer as part of my body, not an invader, and I saw it as something that had to be dealt with so that my body could recover.

I tried to avoid negative thoughts of my body being 'invaded' by cancer, but I did see it as a fight or a race against a condition that I had to be prepared for and participate in to the absolute best of my ability.

Unfortunately, I still have annual tests and check-ups and I have been advised that there is a high likelihood that both the non-Hodgkin lymphoma and the kidney cancers will return. This means I will probably be faced with future decisions about treatments/surgery, which are quite different for each form of cancer.

I have decided that dwelling on whether they return or not is wasted time and energy, and I will deal with the diagnosis either good or bad at the time it happens.

Treatments and medication are constantly improving and evolving and who knows what will be available if or when I need treatment.

There is also the chance that the cancers do not return, and I die of something else, hopefully counting my money in old age.

Whether you are facing a diagnosis or finishing treatment, you always have choices and while you are still breathing you have hope.

I have attempted through this book to provide a general and helpful view of some of the extreme things that a cancer patient may have to deal with during their treatment. By using my experiences, I hope to have shown the deviations from the normal path that may occur during treatments.

I have successfully survived my ordeals to date and am currently thriving and enjoying life despite some of the collateral damage suffered during my various medical experiences.

I am eternally grateful to the treating medical professionals and nursing staff who were involved despite the setbacks that occurred.

Quite simply I would not be alive today if not for their skills and dedication.

My book will hopefully give you some tools to mould your thought processes and actions into strategies that assist you in whatever ordeal you may face.

Final Tip

There are too many things that are out of your control to waste time, effort and energy worrying about what may or may not happen.

Deal with what you have and do your best.

Be prepared to adapt and change as required and never lose your sense of humour.

There is no doubt that what does not kill you makes you stronger.

Good Luck!

Afterword

Coronavirus and how it affects Cancer Patients

While I was writing this book, the world was confronted by a new strain of coronavirus named COVID-19.

Coronavirus encompasses a large group of viruses that cause illnesses.

In this case, the virus appears to have originated from animals and then spread to humans.

Regardless of the origin of the disease, it has decimated the world's population and economies. The outcome of this global human tragedy remains unknown, but there is no doubt that it is the biggest test for a generation of the human race with at best catastrophic outcomes and at worst the deaths of untold people.

While this situation is a global disaster that will continue for some time, my focus is on cancer patients and how they need to change their lives to suit the circumstances, maximise their chances of going through their treatments and surviving.

It is difficult enough to have been diagnosed with cancer (or any other serious disease) at this time, but right now and for some time in the foreseeable future, hospitals, testing facilities and the medical system in general are in crisis mode.

What this means is that only the most urgent of cases will be treated, and patients who do not meet this criteria will have to make the best of their circumstances based on their condition, location and individual needs.

As this spread of disease has prevented movement across and between countries, and in many cases across states and regions, with many people in lockdown or quarantine combined with hospital and emergency departments clogged with COVID-19 protocols, the normal testing, treatment regimens and timetables have been seriously disrupted if not cancelled.

The medical system is adapting quickly to attempt to provide services to their patients but there is no doubt that cancer patients will be experiencing increased anxiety in relation to their condition and treatment.

There is an increased urgency for cancer patients and others with compromised immune systems to practise social distancing, increased cleanliness regimes and to be more vigilant in these difficult times so that they do not succumb to the virus and its dangerous implications.

If you have tests, scans or other pre-treatment appointments scheduled, contact the service providers or medical practitioners and confirm that these will still be proceeding and if not, what strategies need to be adopted until they can be conducted.

The same applies in relation to surgery, radiation or chemotherapy treatments scheduled prior to the COVID-19 crisis as in most countries, only urgent cases are being progressed. You need to know what the criteria is and what to do if you do or do not meet these revised treatment protocols.

The same principles as I have detailed in my book in relation to attitude, self-reliance, positive thinking and meditation and relaxation techniques now more than ever need to be applied to suit this new set of circumstances.

Cancer patients are different from the general population due to the specifics of their condition and the complex and often lengthy periods of treatment required to manage their conditions.

Our current circumstances in many cases will restrict family involvement and support and place many unforeseen hardships on patients and their support networks.

These times will test us all, but the key strategy will be the ability to adapt to the circumstances you are faced with and deal with them in the best possible way.

If you are able to manage your condition during this

difficult time until there is a return to some form of normality, the medical system should be able to wind down their current crisis status and start to treat the backlog of medical cases that have been postponed during the COVID-19 outbreak.

Unfortunately, the new normality may not look much like our previous perception of normality. We can only be aware of the circumstances we are faced with and adapt to and deal with those circumstances to the best of our ability at this stage of the COVID-19 crisis, but who knows what the future may bring.

Summary of Tips

Tip Number 1

If possible, take a family member or support person to the meeting and ask the permission of the medical practitioner to record the meeting. This helps when relaying the information to family or friends and ensures that you have all the information delivered at the time and also allows time to consider the details and consider your options.

Tip Number 2

Once you have the initial diagnosis, research as much information as you can on treatment options, medication and associated side effects specific to your condition and compile questions for your next visit to the medical practitioner treating you.

Tip Number 3

Compile a file including a notebook and keep all your medical information in one place (one or more files) for easy access and reference. Download and recorded information to your PC for backup and place all electronic communications related to your medical issues in one place on your PC and on a backup hard drive if possible.

Tip Number 4

Sometimes medical treatment comes at a cost, but sometimes the cost determines the treatment.

Tip Number 5

Once you get a serious diagnosis, start straightaway on improving your overall health and fitness consistent with your individual personal circumstances and medical condition through diet and exercise and relaxation activities.

Your GP should be able to assist with general advice on these activities before you commence a new or improved exercise and diet regime.

Tip Number 6

If you are unsure of the need for a particular expensive and or invasive test or procedure, raise it with your treating doctor and request an explanation on why it is necessary and what may be some other options.

Tip Number 7

If it hurts, or is not working, or you are uncomfortable, tell somebody, stick up for yourself, ask questions, seek other opinions, get somebody who knows how to do the procedure.

Don't suffer in silence and hope that things will improve on their own.

Always be polite and respectful but firm, and don't forget humour can diffuse many difficult situations.

Tip Number 8

Have faith in your doctor/specialist, and if you don't, seek another opinion and/or referral.

Tip Number 9

Try and find something funny in almost everything that you do, believe me it helps.

The more you feel sad and sorry for yourself the more this feeling will be reflected by others.

Tip Number 10

Dignity, status and modesty quickly become casualties of testing, treatment and Hospitalisation.

Don't worry about walking around a hospital with your gown undone down the back and your bum hanging out, believe me no one cares, they are all the same and it is part of hospital life.

Your appearance and dress while undergoing some of these procedures and treatments is the last thing you should worry about.

Tip Number 11

Work with the nurses and doctors but if things are going badly, identify the problem and have it rectified as soon as possible.

Tip Number 12

Do whatever you can to get moving and stay positive and motivated. Get a buddy and do things together, chat online or talk about your issues, goals and achievements.

Record all of these things in your medical journal.

Tip Number 13

If something is wrong, if your treatment or care is not being administered or is neglected, deal with it, look after your care, don't become a statistic, make some noise!

Tip Number 14

Lack of sleep can be upsetting for spouses and family members also living in the house, and they should be made aware of your discomfort and how you are dealing with it, and how they may be able to help.

Tip Number 15

If you are going to be a number, be number 1.

Tip Number 16

If you are prescribed drugs, conduct your own research into their common side effects and relative contraindications (possible adverse reactions with other drugs, which under certain circumstances may be necessary when the benefit outweighs the risk) and if you are experiencing any of the side effects, contact your GP and/or treating Specialist and discuss your concerns.

Do the research anyway, whether you are experiencing side effects or not so that you can understand the drug/s, its use and possible contraindications.

Tip Number 17

Living through your cancer experience takes attitude, planning and dedication working in conjunction with your medical treatment to get the best results. Planning all the aspects of your treatment, the possible side effects, days when you can and can't exercise, and what you can and cannot achieve are all methods of controlling what you can control and dealing with as best you can the things that you cannot.

Tip Number 18

Reducing fatigue and improving your mental and physical health are positive ways of contributing to the end result.

Tip Number 19

Any exercise is better than none, and although most of us when going through the process have days of despair and sickness, the achievement of small goals and improvements through increased activity levels and sleep patterns can aid recovery much better than the opposite.

Tip Number 20

Enjoy the little things in life for one day you'll look back and realise they were the big things.

Tip Number 21

It is part of recovery to have days of pain and or fatigue and sickness, this is part of the healing process and should be embraced for what it is and not the end of the world.

Tip Number 22

Battling cancer is a life or death fight and should be treated as such, the battle won't be won unless the good fight is fought.

Tip Number 23

Self-talk is important, so removing negative thoughts and catastrophising is something that you and only you can control.

This thought alone becomes a powerful tool.

You can choose to be angry and you can choose to be sad.

You can also choose to be happy and positive.

A simple strategy that can benefit anybody is to trick your brain into a better place.

One of these tricks is to smile and tell yourself that things are good, and you are happy when faced with bad news, pain or feelings of apprehension and anxiety.

By looking at what you are telling yourself, looking at your thinking, at your irrational beliefs and self-defeating attitudes, you can change them to preferences instead of absolute musts.

You can then experience 'normal' stressful reactions.

In other words, you can create healthy tension and thoughts instead of unhealthy distress.

Tip Number 24

Don't blame society, climate change, the Government or bad luck for your circumstances, if you have cancer deal with it and give it your best shot, it will either work or it won't.

Tip Number 25

Imprint some items that remind you of pleasant places and take them with you for all treatments/procedures and medical appointments.

Tip Number 26

The choice of how you view the future is yours and yours alone.

Final Tip

There are too many things that are out of your control to waste time, effort and energy worrying about what may or may not happen.

Deal with what you have and do your best.

Be prepared to adapt and change as required and never lose your sense of humour.

There is no doubt that what does not kill you makes you stronger.

Acknowledgements

I would like to acknowledge the support of my wife, Sandra, daughter Kaitlyn and son Darren who not only cared for me during my many ordeals and put up with my at times erratic behaviour but who gave me a reason to fight the good fight and stay in the world of the living.

My tennis partner Len Yates kept me amused and focused over the years. He also enabled us to keep the tennis going and to set a record of gold medal wins in the Pan Pacific Masters Games that spans over 14 years and will be hard to beat.

It also must be acknowledged that although in this book I identify and explain some quite horrific blunders that have occurred during my various treatments and hospital stays, the medical profession including carers and nursing staff have undoubtedly saved my life and I owe them a huge debt of gratitude.

In particular Dr D. E. McMahon MB BS, my local GP and friend, my haematologist, Dr Greg Seeley MBBS Hons (1st Class), FRCPA FRACP, and my urologist and robotics surgeon, Dr Charles Chabert MBChB, MRCS(Ed), FRACS (Urol), as they have helped me successfully navigate through my medical journey with their dedication and professionalism.

Last but not least I wish to thank my editor Gail Tagarro and designer Helen Christie for their help, wise counsel and technical assistance to get this book to publication.

About the Author

Leigh Bernhardt is a 66-year-old who has enjoyed a successful business and sporting career.

He currently resides on the Gold Coast in Queensland Australia with his wife Sandra Anne. He has two adult children, Kaitlyn and Darren, and two lovely grandchildren, Hudson and Connor.

Leigh still plays competitive golf, tennis and table tennis, exercises regularly and is in remission from two cancers at this stage.

www.ingramcontent.com/pod-product-compliance
Lightning Source LLC
Chambersburg PA
CBHW021902020426
42334CB00013B/446